THE VIEW FROM MY CHAIR

THE VIEW FROM MY CHAIR

From my heart to yours, the softer side of the healthcare profession

Judith M. Stein, RDH

Editor: C. Susan Nunn, csusannunn.com
Cover design: Pro_eBook Covers
Illustrator: John David Stein
Book Interior and E-book Design Amit Dey, amitdey2528@gmail.com

Paperback ISBN: – 978-1-7374338-1-1
eBook ISBN: – 978-1-7374338-0-4

Dedication

These collections of thoughts are humbly dedicated to every past, present and future comrade in the healthcare profession. From my heart to yours, thank you. Thank you for the example you set before me. I stand humbly on your shoulders. Thank you for the compassion, understanding and encouragement you've shared with me. I pray I've shared that forward. Thank you for showing up when you were exhausted, frustrated, jubilant, fearful or any plethora of emotions you might have carried with you. Know and believe you are not alone. You are enough. And you are so worth it!

So, get comfortable and enjoy this simple read. My hope is to fill you up with encouragement, understanding, and if I'm lucky, maybe a sprinkle of enlightenment.

TABLE OF CONTENTS

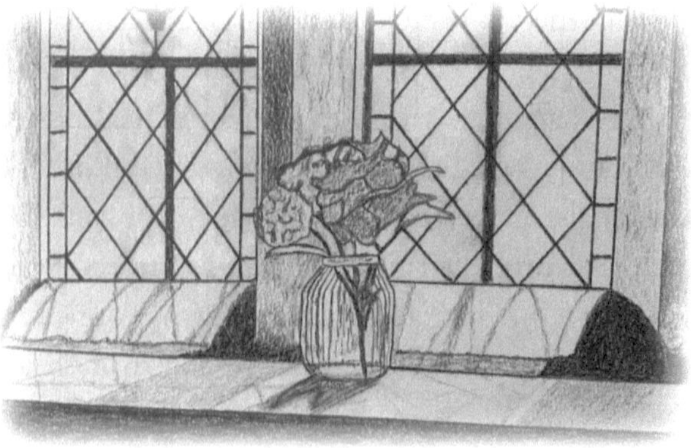

INTRODUCTION

As I arrived to work early one morning, I gazed out my operatory window and realized this was a routine I had been doing for 40 plus years. A flood of questions then rolled through my mind as I allowed my heart to soak up the beauty outside my window. Did I know when I first began my career in healthcare I would still be doing it forty years later? Had I even thought past that moment? Sure, I had been to school, but how many of us change our minds after reality sets in? When I first began, my career was not what it has grown into today. I realize now that as each of us comes to the chair, so to speak, we will incorporate our own values into this career, embracing the changes in the job itself and in ourselves each day.

So, tell me, if someone asked why you were interested in or had already chosen a career in healthcare, what would your answer be? I've often wondered if other health professionals or students experienced a pivotal moment in time that propelled them into their careers. Was there a turning point when you chose to "own" your profession – when you chose to go the distance? For many healthcare professionals, a global pandemic was never on our radar, but now that we have experienced it, did you ever consider riding out something of this magnitude? Could you carry the weight of additional PPE, along with the fear of infection transmission, on your shoulders day after day? Could there have been an emotional incident or financial expectation or circumstantial connection that helped launch you into this profession? What has you curious about exploring this profession? What has kept you in this profession? When exactly did healthcare become your passion? Or has it?

So many questions you may or may not have answers to. That's ok. You could be like me and move from "I have all the answers" to "I have no idea what I'm doing." Then, make another 360 jump from "I love what I do" to "I'm not sure I can make it another day." Seriously. That may sound a bit bipolar and maybe it is, but I don't think it's all that unusual. You see, personally, I believe we'll all have some really great days, some really hard days and a lot of in-between days that make up our career. Join me as I share my thoughts and experiences on how to navigate those days, especially the harder ones.

For me, "hard" started right out of the gate. If I close my eyes, even today, I can still see my naïve 19-year-old self walking to my car after my first day on the job as a dental hygienist, a proud member of the health profession. Forty years ago, a dental hygienist was expected to perform all his or her duties while typically allowed 45 minutes for an average adult and 30 minutes for a child to complete those commitments. Mixed in with those expectations, I would also have to call and confirm every patient on my next day's schedule as well as fill out, by hand, all insurance forms for each patient I served that day. So, if you were in that parking lot, 40 years ago, you'd see my scrawny 19-year-old self walking out to my car wearing an all-white uniform with a plastic smile pasted on my face. That is until I got into my car where the ugly crying started and the tears began to flow.

I was physically and emotionally beat up that first day. I felt like a failure with nowhere to turn. The only thing that got me through the next 12 hours was knowing I was supposed to bring in donuts for my co-workers the next day. I know. Anyone else reading this might wonder about the humor of bringing in donuts to a dental office but I kid you not, it happens. In some ways, thinking about donuts was actually a good distraction for me as I wiped the snot from my nose and drove myself home that day.

I figured I had the next 12 hours to either find a way to gracefully leave a career I had just started or to pull up my big girl pants and get back in the arena. Thankfully, I chose to keep showing up, even if that meant getting my butt kicked for a while. And I am beyond grateful I did so. I cannot tell you how many blessings have been showered over me because of the dental profession. There were challenges too, but the blessings (and donuts) have always won out.

So, let's dig a little deeper into the elements I believe will help you flourish in the healthcare field. To start with, I believe underlying these elements one must become passionate about their career. Ever wonder where such passion is born or how to awaken its pulse again? What gives birth to this unstoppable force that can push through insurmountable obstacles? Today, I feel passion exists in every human but our expression of this desire is as unique to an individual as the composition of our DNA coding. But even if our focus of passion or the expression of this drive cannot be duplicated, I believe you can unleash its potential. With passion, the world is changed. Yes, I believe there is passion in healthcare.

As I look back on my 40-year career as a practicing dental hygienist, I've had to draw from that well of passion endless times. In fact, I've had to re-create my expression of it over and over and over again. What began as a soulful desire to help others through the unknown of dentistry evolved into a mindful expression of service with every patient I've been humbled to work with. I wonder though. Could passion, in its purest form, also be expressed as compassion? If you break the word compassion apart you have the prefix *com* which means with, together or in association with. Place it next to the base word *passion* which means any strongly felt intense emotion, affection or enthusiasm and you have a beautiful marriage. Yes, I do believe passion can walk hand in hand with compassion.

Question is, how does one tap into this union? How do you keep that well of passion/compassion full and ready to spill out onto others around you, as well as yourself? Despite the explosion of external stimuli in our world today, I believe we can slowly unleash the awareness of living more passionately and compassionately, more simply yet abundantly, living more mindfully, more in the moment. With authors like Brene' Brown, Simon Sinek, Sarah Ban Breathnach, Regina Brett, and John Cabot Zin you can drink freely from a source of loving-kindness and encouragement. Today, we can make peace with our past, leave the future where it belongs and live wholeheartedly in the moment.

Forgive me though if I make the expression of this union sound easy. I can honestly share with you that at times my journey towards compassion was a smooth highway. I have also found my way down some very uncomfortable gravel roads. Roads I needed to tread more slowly along during challenging times of my life. For me, I had to make peace with a personal issue early on in my career.

I had no choice. Many of my insecure feelings, as well as empathetic tendencies, all lead back to a simple moment in time that changed my life forever. A moment in time when I led with my mouth and not my brain.

> Backyard baseball. I can still feel the surge of energy pulsing through my scrawny, 10-year-old veins that summer night when some of the neighborhood kids showed up in my backyard. My nickname back then was "twinkle toes" so you can just imagine what a jumpy and giddy 10-year-old I was. Not your typical seasoned athlete either. And having friends over to my backyard was also a pretty big deal. It didn't happen often. To make things even more exciting, I was playing catcher. And you know, to this day, I can still feel the pulse of excitement rushing through me as I began walking towards my field position.
>
> As I mentioned earlier, I was a tad on the smaller side of life, so to be chosen as the catcher was a big deal to me. It's no secret now, but I had no idea what being a catcher even meant. Do the song lyrics, "put me in coach" ring any bells? Well, singing my way onto a baseball field was probably my only hope of playing ball that evening, or so I thought. Sadly, I think my emotions momentarily pushed all the brain

cells out the top of my skull and into the summer night's airflow too. It was such a perfect evening. Not too windy and still enough daylight left to play a few innings. We even had enough players to fill the bases and enough basic equipment to actually get things started. The only thing we didn't have was a lot of time. Or so I thought. So, taking it upon myself to get the game going I ushered someone to the batting position and yelled to the pitcher to throw that ball. And, as I led with my mouth and not my brain, I forgot to step away from the batter and unfortunately caught the bat in my mouth.

You know, thinking back on that moment in time, I don't recall feeling any pain or anger towards anyone except myself. What I do remember was a tightening in my chest, shortness of breath and what I would describe now as a panic episode. I certainly saw a few stars too, just not the kind in an evening's sky. Something else was really wrong when I instinctively brought my hand to my mouth. Lots of oozing, salty-tasting blood, swelling and numbness in my lips and way too much air coming from the anterior section of my front teeth. It only took me a millisecond to realize, this was not good.

This next sprinkling of time still remains a blur to me. I know my family was there and lovingly cared for me, I just don't have specific memory threads of those events. What I vividly remember though, is the moment I went into my bedroom and looked in the mirror. I was completely alone when I removed my hand from my mouth and stared into the mirror. That moment still brings tears to my eyes 50 years later. You see, as a young child, I can honestly say I never put much stock into my looks. I had a short picky haircut, wore a school uniform to school and most days even brushed my teeth. But when I looked into that mirror at that moment and saw a missing front tooth, I just remember an overwhelming need to become invisible. All I wanted to do was disappear. To start shrinking.

Well, I was still struggling to catch my breath which in hindsight probably helped me stay in my moment. You see, even then, focusing on my breath kept me in the moment. Helped me hang onto the fragile thread of reality that I needed to learn to live in. "Just keep breathing Judy and you'll figure something out" were the words I kept repeating in my mind. My little 10-year-old self was having a stare down with my own reflection and sadly, I didn't like what

I saw. I was already learning that if you bring your hand to your mouth while talking, no one can see your teeth or lack of teeth. Looking into my bedroom mirror, I was already trying to see myself as wonderfully made and not permanently broken.

Now, here is the irony of my life, or should I say dichotomy. After that startling moment in front of my bedroom mirror when I wanted to become invisible, my very next thought was, well what am I going to do now? Those thoughts just jolted me out of my head and brought me back to the earth. I could then hear the commotion going on where the telephone was. The phone calls trying to find emergency dental care on a weekend. I also heard excitement when someone found "my tooth." That seemed so cruel to me hearing others rejoice over what I had lost. Obviously, I didn't realize what a blessing that was to have located a piece of the tooth to temporarily re-implant. So, for me, the pivotal moment in time when passion was born that propelled me into the field of dentistry, took place in front of my bedroom mirror at 4940 Lorraine Ave. That moment in time, when invisible me hoped and prayed, I would learn to smile again.

As many of my dear comrades in healthcare will share, my memories of that loss are but a fraction of what true loss feels like. I have, since that moment in time, lived through many life challenges, struggles and tragedies. I could never compare what happened to me when I was 10 years old to losing a loved one to cancer at age 45 or watching my children go through very painful life experiences. But it was a significant event in my life that changed me forever. For me, what I lost at the moment in time cannot compare to what I found. I believe my mind, soul and body began an evolution towards living and working more compassionately. Today, I attribute my overactive empathy chromosomes to the way other health professionals treated me during the multitude of dental procedures I endured. I can now intimately testify to you that when someone cares what they are doing the experience is completely different than that of someone just going through the motions. There is such a big difference!

So here lies the impetus for this book. The softer side of healthcare. Yes, there truly is a softer side to our beloved career. A side not always nurtured in practice or graded upon in school yet I believe is most responsible for successful career experiences, the development of longevity, of lifelong learning, of stamina and the deep passion to serve others in this profession. Whether you are considering a career in healthcare, beginning your career or are a veteran healthcare provider, I want to offer suggestions from the "other side." No, not the dark side, the softer side. The side that needs to integrate all the technical and academic information with the ability to connect compassionately with patients and yourself. I've spent 40 years in a profession that I am still passionate about. I'd like to share with you some of the fun and simple tips I've integrated into my career. Some of these I stumbled upon, some of them I dug myself out of a ditch from, and some of the ideas just flowed naturally. Join me, I will be sharing from my heart, the softer side of me.

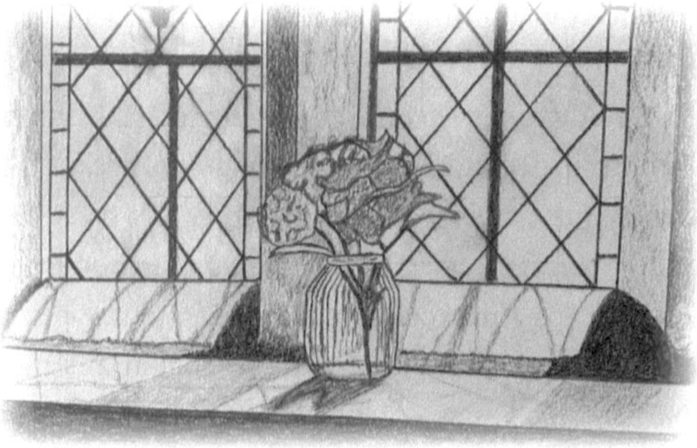

Begin at the Beginning

"Though no one can go back and make a brand new start, anyone can start from now, and make a brand new end." [1]

The words, "Though no one can go back and make a brand new start, anyone can start from now, and make a brand new end" inspire me every day. These words give me hope. Today, I truly believe I have the power to

[1] Bard, Carl. http://www.finestquotes.com/select_quote-category-New%20Beginnings-page-0.htm

begin my day over at any time. In fact, there are days when I don't wait until the end before I begin again. We've all had those kinds of days. Where you seem to be running behind from the start. You mismanage a situation or find yourself dealing with a personal conflict. You might find your pulse racing, temper rising or any other number of bodily reactions. Whatever the cause, know there is a cure to helping turn your day around. And yes, my friend, you can make the decision to do just that at any moment. And trust me, I have. So what's my secret? For me, it's my breath. I know. You're wondering if it could really be that simple. Well, let's find out. Why don't you join me in a generous inhale and soulful exhale as we continue unpacking this concept?

Until I tapped into the power of my breath, I moved through life like a plow horse. Steady yet with blinders on. Whether I was at work or home, I would put my head down and forge forward. Have I mentioned my four children? Have I mentioned almost 40 years in the dental profession? Sadly, moving through life like a plow horse was the only dance I knew the steps to. My mind, body and soul were taking a beating while I kept plowing along. I often missed simple solutions that were right in front of me. I often missed precious moments that I know I can't get back.

Thankfully, after attending a Mindfulness Class in 2016, I now approach life very differently. Today, I choose to stay connected to the mindful awareness of my breath.

I now have a constant resource to tap into whenever I need to steady myself or to begin again. So, what does this look like in my life? What could it look like in yours? For me, it's simple. I use the awareness of my breath to help me stay in the moment, to refocus, to calm down, and to start over if necessary. I mindfully breathe in and out. Noticing how my breath moves through my nostrils. How my stomach and lungs expand as well. And the beautiful thing about this technique is that you can tap into it anytime, anywhere. This precious resource is always available to you.

I also need quiet, meditative moments to begin my day and sometimes to help me start over as well. You may not connect to meditation, and that is completely acceptable. Believe me, the world would be very bland if it were filled with only my quiet personality types. But being part of a profession where we interface intimately, both physically and emotionally, eight-plus hours of the day, I believe it is vital we discover a method of attaining serenity to start our day, to stay in our day and to even bring closure to our day. Trust me on this point, life will get messy but that doesn't mean you can't learn to rise above the challenges. Stay with me. Let's dig a little deeper.

Let's get to know a little more about ourselves. How do we interact in the world around us? Where and how do we tap into this energy source? How can we refill it? One resource available to help you answer those questions is a simple personality assessment. Have you ever done

one? If you'd like to complete a personality assessment to discover more about yourself there are a gambit of tests offered today. The Meyer-Briggs Type Indicator[2] created by Isabel Briggs Myers, and her mother, Katharine Briggs, is one such method to help you identify your personality type and how you interact in the world around you. There are many other variations that will provide you more personal awareness such as the online Enneagram tests. Are you a Type 2, Wing 3? A Type 7, Wing 8? Why not treat yourself to uncovering this information about your style of expression. You can easily go online to begin this journey. But, if all you have now are a few moments, consider the following simple questions to help you begin to identify your personal needs and style of meeting them.

Are you someone who feels energized around other people? After working a full day, do you seek out other people to be with? Do you like more playful, energetic music? Do you drive with music playing in the car? Do your choices of physical activity include Zumba and other group activities? Some may classify you as an extrovert, an outgoing gregarious person. Honor this and seek out these activities to help keep your tank full.

Are you someone who becomes energized with a few moments of peace and quiet? After working a full day do you prefer moments of quiet to regain your composure, fill up your energy tank? Are you someone who prefers

2 http://www.myersbriggs.org/my-mbti-personality-type/mbti-basics/

quieter styles of music? Would your physical activity choices include yoga or walking? These characteristics may find you expressing yourself more as an introvert, a person more likely to turn inward. Again, honor this and seek out those types of behaviors to feed your soul.

Whatever set of scenarios you identify with, or if you find yourself an amalgamation of both, begin by acknowledging what you need, accept your style and then totally embrace it. It was only by trial and error that I uncovered how I moved in the world around me. Turns out I'm not a purest. I am a combination of both introversion and extroversion. I am what is known as an ambivert. An ambivert is one whose personality type is a beautiful blend of both extroversion and introversion. This totally explains why I love and treasure quiet, meditative time but also love being with people. Go figure, I never had to choose one personality camp. I could move between the two. I only needed to become aware and identify how I moved in the world around me.

Educating yourself and learning more about all personality characteristics could be a huge blessing for your career, your personal life and everyone you come in contact with. Think about it. Whether you are dealing with a family member, a co-worker or a patient, when you better understand how they move in the world, your interactions will be more genuine, less judgeful and more impactful.

Personally, with every patient I work with, I begin the appointment by noticing their behaviors while I am escorting them back to my operatory. Are they quiet? Do I sense a more thoughtful shy demeanor, a more cautious posture? If those answers are yes, I may be dealing with a person with more introverted tendencies. Maybe your patient is extremely talkative, much more expressive. They seem to want to engage you in conversations versus quiet moments. These expressions are more typical of an extroverted person by nature. Could there be any signs of anxiety?

Whatever personality characteristics or behaviors your patient is displaying, your observations can begin to build a solid foundation for your relationship. You could more easily connect with them or slightly adapt your behavior to ease the relationship. You could also choose to mirror their behaviors or detach from them with kindness. Whatever choice you make please keep in mind that observing behavior is not a free pass to judge anyone. You are only collecting information in order to better connect with your patient, co-worker, friend or family member. I strongly caution you not to judge or categorize anyone. Remember, we are all a beautiful blend of fluid behaviors. We need never put anyone in a box, including ourselves.

So, begin at the beginning and get to know more about yourself and others around you. Completely embrace these discoveries and work towards fostering whatever brings you inner peace. If you are already on this journey, I encourage you to keep moving forward. If you are just starting out, be gentle with yourself. Remember, you can begin your day, or start your day over, at any time. Never forget the essence of your breath. Allow yourself the time every day to receive the priceless gifts of peace and serenity. Your personal and professional life will never be the same. So go for it! Start now, and make a brand-new end.

Reflection:

Do you identify as an extrovert, introvert or ambivert? Journal what activities would best support your personality style and consider plugging them into your daily living. Remember, awareness can lead to action. And you're worth it!

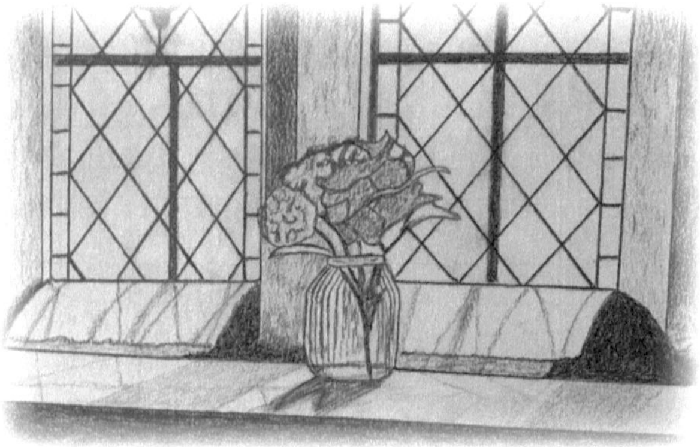

Gratitude

Gratitude is my game changer. My "go-to" when I find myself struggling with any number of situations going on around or within me. Seriously. I can't tell you how many times I have found myself in a challenging situation, personal or professional, that I had to lean deeply into gratitude to pull myself out. What others believed as "only seeing life through rose-colored glasses" was actually a skill I had worked very hard to attain. Trust me, I don't wear those glasses 24/7. I just keep them close by and know when I need to put them on.

I think it's important we pause here. Although I wholeheartedly believe in the practice of gratitude, I now know that gratitude doesn't cancel out other feelings, nor should it. You can't tell someone that being grateful for the home they live in will take away all the painful feelings of a divorce. Gratitude just doesn't work that way. For me, the practice of gratitude helps to see what else is going on around me, not just the struggle I am in. Gratitude helps keep the shackles of self-pity and victimhood from taking my soul prisoner too.

Early on in my career, I wasn't as focused on gratitude as I could have been though. Sadly, I was all about trying to be perfect. I don't even like typing that word anymore, but almost 40 years ago I was all about trying to get it perfectly right, all the time. Don't get me wrong, as I've said before, health professionals are trained to seek and achieve excellence when working with patients. What was missing in my life was how to deal with my imperfections, when I didn't get them perfect. Looking back, this probably wasn't a skill-set my college instructors could have put into their curriculum, but I sure needed it. I needed to learn how to use an ultrasonic scaler and also how to shake off feelings of shame when I didn't get it right. I needed to learn how to work professionally with patients but not to bring their negative attitudes home with me. Maybe all I really needed was to grow up and stop taking myself so seriously but I just wasn't in that space yet.

Thankfully, as I have pushed through my professional and personal challenges, I have come to realize the importance of kindness, compassion and an attitude of gratitude when dealing with my life struggles. For me, it all circles back to looking for the positive in every situation, learning from those experiences and again, to stop taking myself so seriously. Today, these life skills are what frees me up to continue learning, growing and moving gently in the world around me. Now, when I'm at work, I bring my gratitude glasses with me and attempt to play a more thoughtful soundtrack of encouragement in my mind.

Some of my self-talk now includes:

> I am running 20 minutes behind because of an unexpected need my patient presented with **but** my next patient was notified of this circumstance and is politely waiting for me. If this patient needs to be rescheduled though, I will follow up with a personal note of apology.
>
> My co-worker is on the struggle bus today **but** I have the next eight hours to offer him/her kindness and understanding. Always keep in mind we never truly know the struggle another person is going through. Don't live in the space of judgment. As the saying goes, "when you point one finger, there are three pointing back at yourself."

> Speaking of pointing, my employer has pointed out an area I need to improve upon that I already feel competent in **but** I choose not to feel self-defeated. Rather, I look with fresh eyes at the situation and see what and where I can make changes. I am so grateful to work for someone who cares about my professional development!
>
> I am physically struggling to move with additional PPE needed due to the Coronavirus Pandemic, **but** this equipment is needed to keep myself, my family members, team members and patients safe. After a brief internal pity party, I begin to realize that although my body temperature at work is elevated, the new air purifiers help circulate and cool the air around me. I also work in a space with windows that can be opened to bring in the fresh air. I am beyond grateful for the wisdom and perseverance my employer has to attain all needed PPE to help keep me safe.

Ready for some more examples of how I rock those gratitude glasses? Let's jump back in time to the year 1987. I wonder if you can relate to the physical, mental and emotional exhaustion of new parenthood. This was a big one for me. I had happily been riding the "I love my life and my job" train for a while. Then, when the birth of my first child came along, a child I had longed for, I was expecting to "carry on as usual" after her birth. I had bought into the world's philosophy that "I could have it all." Parenthood and career could easily be bundled together. Well, it wasn't that easy for me. It is for others and my heart sings for every parent who's had an easier transition. But for me, it wasn't. After an unexpected surgical delivery, I was so completely focused on the challenges of my medical recovery and motherhood that I couldn't see the possibilities. I needed to dust off my rose-colored glasses but I had somehow misplaced them. It wasn't until I had a significant shift in attitude that I became successful in balancing both motherhood and career. I began to focus more on gratitude and less on my deficit. So, what did this look like for me?

> I missed my daughter terribly while I was at work **but** she was cared for by loving daycare providers. My baby wasn't sleeping through the night for nine months **but** she only woke once and went right back to sleep. Returning to work after my daughter was born was difficult **but** in doing so helped provide a home, food and other necessities for my family. My physical body did not look or feel the same as before birth **but** it was strong enough to have given birth to a beautiful daughter and return to work. When I decided to cut back to part-time employment it meant fewer dinners out

> and name-brand clothing **but** in doing so I was able to spend more time with my daughter and husband.

Looking back, I am so thankful I found my gratitude glasses once again. It wasn't easy and it didn't happen overnight but eventually, I began to see light in my world again. I heard the full symphony of laughter in my child's voice. I saw the pinkish-orange of a sunset and felt the joy in accomplishing a challenging task at work once again. I do believe the practice of gratitude will look different for every person on this planet though but I wonder if the results will be similar. If so, maybe we'll all begin seeing life's big beautiful picture and not stay hyper-focused on our challenges. And as author Brene' Brown shares "There is no joy without gratitude.[3]" Choose to *begin at the beginning* with gratitude. Choose joy. Just don't lose your glasses.

Reflection:

List 5 areas of gratitude in your life. Consider purchasing a spiral notebook to capture these gratitude thoughts every day. Do this, because you're worth it!

[3] https://www.azquotes.com/quote/1248167

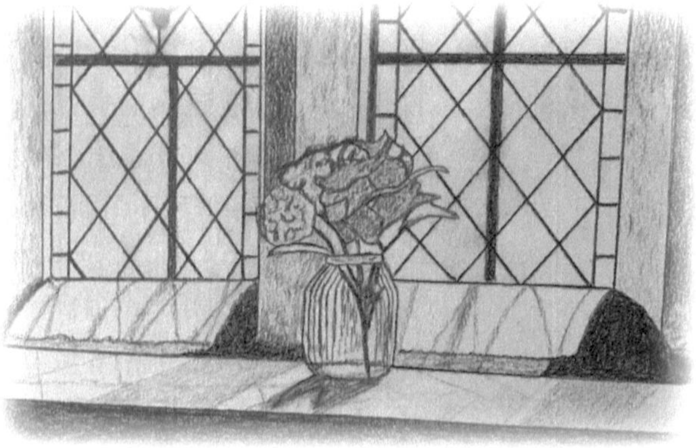

Stay On Top of Your Game But in Your Own Pond

I can still recall the moment I heard the phrase "It's ok to get your ducks in a row but not cool to line-up anyone else's." Maybe another way of saying this is to "keep your nose on your own face." Just think about those two phrases for a minute. OK. Let's get brave. Let's be honest. Can you identify with those behaviors or know someone else who does? Sadly, even with my best intentions, I had been known to jump ponds on a whim causing unnecessary stress, tension and a few waves in the world around me. How about you? Have you ever found yourself telling someone else how to "line up their ducks" versus taking care of your own? Have you ever put your nose into a conversation you were not invited to? Again, been there, done that and have a wardrobe full of tee-shirts to prove it.

Well today, I am so grateful to be aware of this character defect. I have now begun to create healthier boundaries and relationships in my professional and personal life. I'd like to share how applying these concepts has truly liberated me. How living, learning and growing in my own pond has brought back so much joy in my life. So, on that note, get your swimsuit on. Who cares what we look like! Come, join me as I share how I get my own ducks in a row, keep them in some semblance of order, all while giving other ducks the dignity to swim in their own ponds.

For me, lining up my own ducks begins with the pursuit of my personal and professional best. That expression is most evident while I am sharpening my technical skills, stretching my base of knowledge and then sharing those gifts with others. How does all this play out? What does it look like in practical terms? Well, for me, it's simple. I begin by purposing to read at least one dental-related article per week and to also continue my personal reading routines as well. Sound boring? Trust me, it really isn't. When you're looking after your own ducks, you can decide where you'd like to focus your attention. There is freedom swimming in your own pond.

In today's world of social media, it is even easier to receive continuing education information online. These sources can help your ducks learn to swim strongly, confidently and even dodge some seaweed along the way. Between Twitter, Facebook and who knows what next Social Media craze, you can link into many reliable healthcare sites that offer access to current insights and knowledge. Personally, I am a big fan of our professional magazines that offer the latest health profession updates. Whatever your preferred learning style is, make lifelong learning your passion. This simple habit will help keep you aware of challenges as well as trends in the healthcare arena.

This routine can also provide you with the tools and confidence to present the most knowledgeable treatment plan to your patients. Perpetual learning can also show you where your weaknesses are and areas where growth exists. But isn't that still learning? Yes, I believe it is! And never forget to make friends with your local library too. Our libraries still hold the keys to so many doors of opportunity. And for me, it's one of my "happy places." I love the level playing field a library offers every patron. Regardless of your age, gender, sexual orientation or socioeconomic status everyone is treated fairly. Everyone is allowed to drink freely from the library's pond of knowledge.

From your personal homecare routine to your work routines, I cannot emphasize enough how vital it is to keep things balanced and in proper working order. For me, keeping "my ducks in a row" at work begins when I hone my instruments every single morning. I can go through my daily instrument setups in under 10 minutes. And those 10 minutes are priceless! Just try it.

Keeping my ducks in a row at home is prioritizing my prayer, meditation, exercise and family time. I've learned to pause before I say "yes" to a request. Many times, I can still help, but pausing allows me to look at all my ducks to see if any are sinking, slowing down or simply just needing to rest. And it's ok to rest, to slow down. Sometimes those simple actions can help you stay afloat while you tread water. Remember, resting doesn't mean quitting. It just means you are catching your breath. Pausing. Allowing yourself the chance to check in on your ducks and address their needs before you start swimming again.

I'm afraid we can't ignore how our personal and professional routines were dramatically affected by the Covid 19 global pandemic. Our ponds and ducks all took a beating. There was no denying that our work protocols had to be re-evaluated and significantly changed. Each department needed to discover solutions, implement them and be willing to continually adapt to this crisis. I was extremely fortunate to be led through this event by someone who encouraged cross-over thinking yet gave each department the dignity to solve their challenges. For example, I believe it would have been inappropriate to stick my nose into the department that handles the new protocol for patient check-in. If I was asked for advice or feedback, I shared it. Otherwise, I respected their solutions. If I had a question, I asked it, but I did not tell others how to do their job.

This behavior went both ways. When other departments communicated that they would not be utilizing aerosol-producing ultrasonics until we had a more high-powered evacuation system, they were totally supported by the entire office. We worked together, without micro-managing each other's efforts. No one had to swim alone but we certainly respected each other's waterways.

So, keep your swimsuit handy. Get to know the pond you swim in. Personally, I see mine loaded with lily pads, turtles, fish and even some cattails near the shoreline. Don't be afraid to invite others over to swim with you but make sure you ask before you visit their pond. I truly believe every challenge, today and in the future, can spring forth opportunities to grow and rise even stronger. And as we travel down these waterways of life, I promise to swim alongside you, as we, the healthcare community and the world, become a rising phoenix, not a sitting duck.

Reflection:

What professional and personal obligations belong in someone else's pond and not your own? Once you identify these items, begin detaching from them. Detaching with kindness and concern, not abandonment or hatred. After you've identified what ducks don't belong in your pond, begin focusing on what is in your pond. Fine-tune those skills. Own your strengths and build on your weaknesses. You won't regret this and you're worth it!

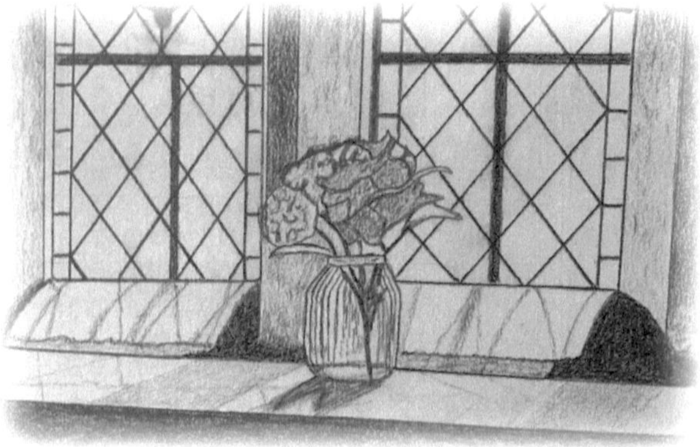

It's Not All About Me? Really?

"Dental Diva" is a term I hope is never used to describe me. If I'm completely honest though, and willing to evaluate my personal and professional behavior, I must ask myself, do I project that attitude into the world around me, including my workspace? Do my insecurities and fears give birth to isolation instead of companionship? Again, so many questions that couldn't possibly be answered on a clinical evaluation form or written test while in school. Questions, however, that need to be addressed, even if the process is a bit uncomfortable. I promise you though, you won't regret the journey from diva to delightful. Trust me, it's really just a few more vowels and consonants to get there.

I personally think there is a fine line to navigate between confidence and superiority. Yes, we've all been through very rigorous professional training. This is where many of our professional attitudes and expectations are formed and shaped. We are under constant evaluation from our professors to project an air of confidence. However, without an element of genuine compassion, an attitude of "I want it all, I can do it all. I am responsible for it all" may seep through our skin, eventually spilling over into our workspace. This behavior is certainly not confined to the healthcare profession though. It can sneak into other professional and volunteer arenas as well. But hang on, it gets better. There is hope.

But first, time for true confessions. When I courageously began to evaluate the effect I had on other co-workers, I started to realize I was projecting an attitude of superiority without even meaning to. I wanted it all! I wanted to learn everything, practice everything, and suggest everything at every staff meeting. When I became crazy on fire for dentistry though, I began to notice fewer interactions from co-workers. I, without meaning to, began to feel isolated from my co-workers and I was ultimately the one responsible for this. The more I was rapidly pushing my ideas out there, the more that action seemed

WHAT READERS ARE SAYING

While this book contains loads of advice for new healthcare and established healthcare professionals, it is also for anyone who wants to experience continuous improvement as a human being. Take this journey with Judy and find ways to be a better person. It's what the world needs from all of us.

~ Teresa M O'Brien,
author of four self-help books

"As a patient of Judy's for nearly 20 years I can attest that she embodies compassion for her patients and love for her profession. You can hear it and feel it when you're in her chair–the concern, empathy, curiosity, gratitude, joy, and more. This book beautifully details how she continually looks inside herself to ensure every patient that sits in her chair experiences that same cared-for feeling. The reflection questions at the end of each chapter are a chance to use her story to reflect on your own. I highly recommend this book for any healthcare professional looking to reignite their passion for their work and move beyond simply clinical care to genuinely compassionate care for patients."

~Rachel A. Larimore, Ph.D.

to push others away from me. Instead of drawing others into my space, I was alienating them.

Quick pause here. I am not, under any circumstance suggesting you become or remain a person that others take advantage of. Absolutely not! Your thoughts, your concerns are critical to the world we live in. I won't tolerate a bully nor would I ever want you to. But with the pendulum of confidence swinging in many directions, including my own personality style, I believe it's vital we discover the happy middle point. Recently I stumbled upon the author, Brene' Brown's phrase, "Don't shrink, don't puff up, just stand your sacred ground."[4] Isn't that beautiful? I truly believe that simple phrase has the potential to help everyone move more comfortably, more cohesively and more compassionately in our workplace and the world around us.

So, how does one move through life not shrinking, not puffing up but standing in their own sacred space? How can you blend an air of confidence with genuine compassion and not wear a tiara? How can you fuse your own personality style with your co-workers and with the overall success of our healthcare profession? For me, it began to happen when I realized it really isn't all about me. I work with an amazing team! Have the courage to be your own enthusiastic self. Be passionate about healthcare, just don't squash others in the process.

[4] https://www.goodreads.com/author/quotes/162578.Bren_Brown?page=10

It is also important to note that each co-worker holds a piece of valued knowledge that I need to show respect towards during staff meetings and professional conversations throughout the day. I don't have to agree with the shared information, but I do need to respectfully acknowledge that input. A phrase like "you might be right" can quickly diffuse a heated discussion without having to agree or disagree with the person you are in a dialog with.

I also realize that the following statement may sound too trite to even mention, but I believe that each team member holds a piece of the daily schedule. My patient is no more important than the patient with the dental assistant or dentist. We are all in this together! Each co-worker also holds a piece of their personal best. We all influence the goal of practicing and delivering excellence so who am I to believe it must revolve around me. Become a person who builds others up when their ideas are shared, instead of overpowering and limiting the conversation to only your perspective.

I invite you to join with me as I continue to celebrate the amazing healthcare field we are privileged to be a part of. Bring your passions and enthusiasm to every aspect of your career, just leave the tiara at home. Better yet, why not share a little glitz and glamour with your co-workers. Could you just imagine how much we could ALL shine together?

Reflection:

What actions could you take to ensure all co-workers and family members are respected? Could you offer a shout-out at a staff meeting highlighting a co-worker's achievement? Could you take a family member out for some one-on-one time to really focus on that person? Could you be known as an encourager rather than the dominator? Just think of simple ways you could help the light from others shine as bright as yours. Go for it because you're worth it!

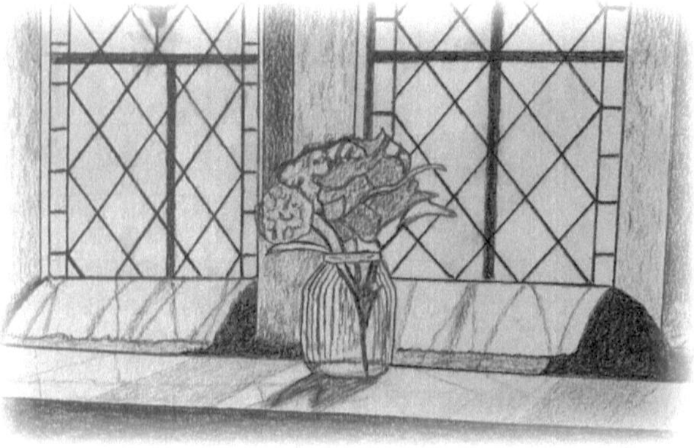

Fun on Fridays!

I had the privilege of working with a wonderful human who, in my humble opinion, when practicing, was an exemplary healthcare professional. A person who brought their best effort to every interaction and procedure she encountered. Maybe you already know someone like this. Maybe your healthcare superhero is actually a patchwork of people, behaviors and styles that when pieced together make one awe-inspiring human. Maybe you can even see yourself in that vision. Maybe you're still on a journey of discovery. Either way, I'd like to share my thoughts and experiences with the hope that something will resonate with you. If nothing connects though, just keep searching. I believe you will eventually find your career superhero/heroes to learn and grow from without putting anyone on a pedestal.

For me, I've had the honor of working with many incredible healthcare professionals. There just happens to be one that stands out to me, at this time in my life. Someone who still occupies space in my mind and heart. Someone who took me almost 15 years into my career to meet. Until that happened, I had often heard other healthcare professionals comment that she was brilliant, colorful, dependable, friendly, and very engaging. Her patients loved her too. It's not that anyone was gossiping about her either. She just had a very solid reputation. For me, even before I met her, I knew I wanted to learn from her. Truthfully, some days, I just wanted to be her.

So guess what I discovered when I finally began working with this amazing human? Yes, she was absolutely brilliant and an expert in her field. She was dependable, friendly, a great communicator and a wonderful team player. But what I also discovered that I believe was the key to her success, was her gift of flexibility and the fun way she expressed that attribute. Flexibility and fun do not mean she was a pushover. Just the opposite. She knew and wanted the best for her patients and every team member she worked with. She would go to bat for any vulnerable soul needing a champion. She also knew which battles to choose and did so with dignity, grace and yes, fun! Even the way she dressed brightened every space she entered. Her color choices were bright and bold, compared to my comfort shades of neutrals. Somehow, she just brought balance to the world around her. Not by making her presence seem overpowering but rather by adding colorful energy to everyone she served and worked with.

For me, the first lesson I learned from her was yes, we could have fun while administering our absolute best at work. This was new to me. I tended to take my work so seriously. I "worked hard" (remember that plow horse) but seemed to forget I could "play hard" too. Well, thankfully she and I shared a few Fridays together. I got to witness her having "fun on Fridays." We never did anything different on the outside, but her positive inner attitude was infectious and made everyone around her happy. I saw her choose happiness instead of grumpiness over and over and over again. Even if she had to remind the Doctor she was waiting for a patient exam, her attitude was positive and understanding. She never put others on the defensive or projected judgment. It appeared that she truly understood everyone was doing their best at that moment in time. She saw the big picture of keeping her serenity even during challenging moments. This amazing human stayed flexible which seemed to feed into her positive attitude. She, without knowing it, became a shining star in my professional career. She became one of my career superheroes.

I wonder if you have a Superhero or North Star in your professional life. Someone who has pointed the way, modeled to you excellent professional and personal behavior? Who are your mentors, co-workers, family members and or friends that have shown you how to smile, how to be your best, how to have fun, how to stay flexible? Who are the people in your life that challenged you as well as encouraged you? I was professionally blessed to have worked with many incredible dental practitioners all of whom I am genuinely grateful for. I've spent most of my professional career just soaking up information, honing dental techniques and serving others. I could never have experienced such a rewarding occupation/ministry had it not been for those that went before me, walked alongside me and the many who will follow.

On a personal note, I was also significantly blessed to have known another beautiful soul who helped light my way forward. She was a devoted daughter, amazing wife, a wonderful mother, respected employee of our local newspaper who also happened to have lost her sight in her early thirties. What she wasn't though was a person with a disability. Although she had vision challenges that labeled her legally blind that never stopped her from living her best life. She didn't see herself with limitations, rather, she saw life as an adventure. My friend had a lovely and generous way of not taking herself too seriously either. Laughter was always good medicine in her life, and she shared that recipe with everyone she met.

There are so many other humans who have added to the galaxy of stars in my life. I hope that you too will recognize the light in your own soul and seek to shine even brighter. Who knows, you may already be a superhero in training. Maybe you're like me and still gleaning from others. Maybe you're a little bit of both. So, go ahead. Have some fun on Fridays. Have some fun every day! Don't be afraid to be flexible. Don't take yourself too seriously. I believe you can achieve incredible professional and personal satisfaction without having everything go perfectly your way. You can have fun and spread that joy to everyone you encounter. I believe you will find your professional and personal relationships much more enjoyable. Just remember to let your inner beauty shine through you. I think you'll be pleasantly surprised when that light boomerangs right back your way.

Reflection:

Consider taking a moment to recognize and then thank the "North Stars," the superheroes in your life. A small note, a quick text, a simple phone call or as Charles Caleb Colton[5] states, "Imitation is the sincerest form of flattery"[6] Learn to develop the skills in those you most admire because you are worth it!

[5] https://www.goodreads.com/author/quotes/901497.Charles_Caleb_Colton

[6] https://www.brainyquote.com/quotes/quotes/c/charlescal203963.html

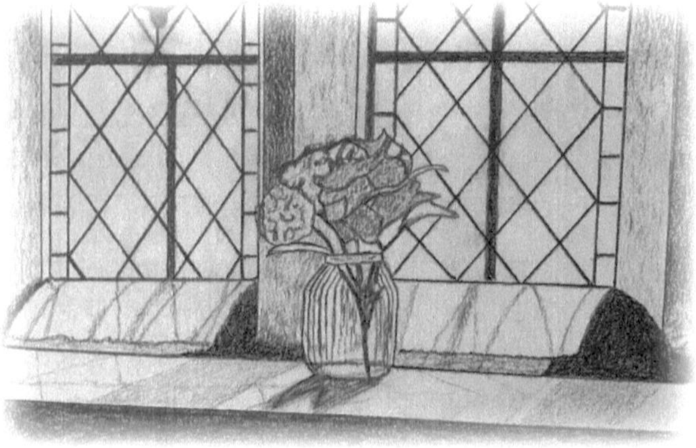

HIPAA Before It Was HIPAA

I can't tell you how many times I've misspelled or mispronounced the acronym HIPAA while typing or speaking on this topic. In fact, there are still moments when I want to say or type HIPPO, with a smile on my face, of course, instead of HIPAA. I mean no disrespect, just wanting to set a more cheerful undertone for a sometimes flat topic. So I will dare you stay in the car with me as we cruise down the HIPAA Highway. You see, long before the acronym HIPAA, **Health Insurance Portability**

and Accountability Act,[7] became part of our healthcare vocabulary I believe many health professionals knew, deep down, of the critical need for this confidentiality code. I personally believe we all have an ethical obligation to guard our patient's records with great reverence and security. In my opinion, following the core values established by HIPPA is basic to survival and success in any career and in your personal life as well. Stay with me though. This won't be a lecture. Just keep your seatbelt buckled.

In my early twenties, way before HIPAA was a part of our healthcare vocabulary, I needed routine blood work performed at a hospital. As I was in queue for my turn to have blood drawn, I looked up to see a 3ft X 5ft whiteboard directly in front of me. Most of the medical procedures and names written on this board meant nothing to me. Unfortunately, right in broad daylight, there was also the name of my neighbor and her personal health information right in front of my eyes. Just seeing this information made me feel like an intruder. It was so awkward. It's not that I could leave either. By now, I had a tourniquet wrapped around my arm and a needle drawing blood from my veins. But what I did choose to do at that moment was to look away and dismiss what I saw. To this day, I can honestly say, that information has never been shared with another person. I also believe, everyone

---

[7] http://www.hhs.gov/ocr/privacy/index.html U.S. Department of Health & Human Services

attached to that event was doing their best. Thankfully today, those whiteboards of confidential information no longer exist in healthcare settings. We now know better, therefore, we do better.

So, will you too become the keeper of confidences? Are you willing to remove any unsecured whiteboards in your area of influence? Whether you like it or not, this honor of keeping confidences will become part of your profession. No matter how small or how significant you think shared information is, it is still to be guarded. I encourage you to embrace this privilege. Guard this honor and guard your mouth. Have you heard the phrase "what happens here, stays here?" Applying that philosophy to events in Las Vegas is much more exciting than what is exchanged in your professional world, but I believe is far more critical. What is shared between you and your patient must be dealt with within the walls of your workspace? If you need to report concerns, report them to appropriate professional sources. If you need to refer your patient, make the necessary confidential referral notes. Do not, however, discuss patient information unless you are seeking professional support. I've even had to bite my tongue when wanting to "share" something with a co-worker. My golden rule is, if it's not kind, necessary, or truthful, keep your mouth closed. Let your co-workers know how you feel about this issue. And trust me, actions will speak louder than words.

I also encourage you to evaluate how much you share with your patients while working with them. I love the personal touch many health professionals have given me. I do not, however, like to hear the constant chatter of a personal nature while someone is working with me. I learned this early on in my career and I'm sure many of you can testify to the same reaction when someone is sharing way too much information with you. It seems to set off a red flag in my gut. I begin to question how focused they are on the work being performed. I also begin to wonder how trustworthy they are with my information if they are sharing way too much of theirs. Granted, if anyone is nervous and is giving you cues to talk them through the procedure, please do so. If they are not nervous though, respect their time and space. Offer them moments of peace and quiet while you work. Create a nurturing environment in your workspace. Serenity is priceless.

Trust me, you truly can live and work in the same community. You can go home to your family even with the knowledge of personal information that must remain confidential. I'd like to share with you three simple words of wisdom from a hospice home director who provided training for me in 2008. He encouraged me to "bless and release." To always do my best. Then, bless and release. This simple phrase has helped me manage many of the privileges and burdens built into my career. To know when to call in additional professional support or to make necessary referrals but not to bring that information home or into the community. Bless and release, my friend. Bless and release.

Reflection:

If you don't have a designated HIPAA employee in your office, take a moment to visit the CDC website on HIPAA compliance to shore up your knowledge on this policy. Capture any thoughts or ideas that you would like to see implemented in your office setting. Take a continuing education class on this topic. Be brave and share your concerns! Nothing changes if nothing changes. And you, my friend, are worth it!

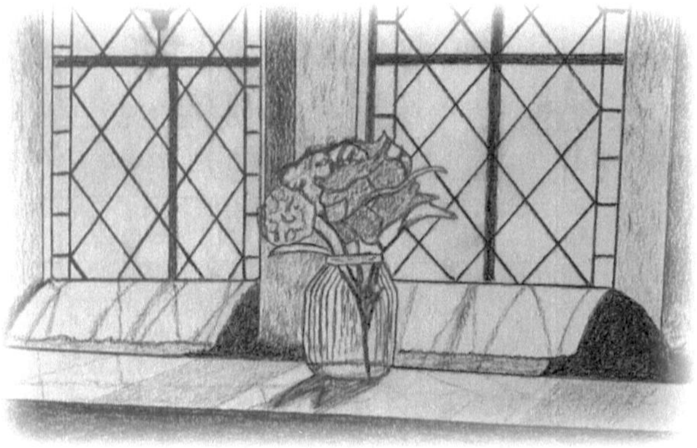

True Confessions – Found Freedom

Some time in your personal life or your professional career, you will need to make peace with your past. I'm not recommending you live in your past, or even make a habit of re-visiting it very often. In fact, I've heard it said that it's ok to look backward, just be careful not to stare. What I'm really trying to promote is that you do not let your past define or own you. Allow every learning experience to bless you and the others you serve. And trust me, nothing in life is ever wasted if we're willing to learn from it.

Sound like a lot of babbling? Well, truth is, I'm doing a pretty good job deflecting you from what I really need to share. So here goes. As you already know, I am a devoted member of the healthcare profession. Inside that profession, I would hope my knowledge and experience in oral care complements other health modalities. So, to share with you that I was a cigarette smoker while in college may or may not surprise you, but it still brings shame to me today just admitting it. Today what I'd like to share with you, however, is not my shame but instead my gratefulness for being an ex-smoker (emphasis on the ex) and how I share that piece of knowledge with others.

Today I am truly liberated from the bondage of cigarette smoking. I also support others who suffer from addiction challenges as well. The freedom I found when I quit smoking, the release of casting judgment on others and the return of my personal health were only a sprinkling of blessings I now possess and share with others. Was it easy? No, it wasn't! Was it worth it? Strong yes! Although I've given birth to 4 children, encountered emergency leg surgery and the removal of my right kidney I still believe quitting smoking was one of the hardest things I've ever done. I was humbled and empowered all in the same breath. And thankfully, today my breath is clean, clear and full of endless possibilities. Because of my journey, I'd like to believe I can more lovingly hold space for others battling addictions, and that, my friends, is priceless.

It did take several years before I felt comfortable and confident sharing this part of my life though. I was very choosey with this information as I suggest you are as well. Trust yourself. You will know who and when to share your personal challenges with. For me, I look for signs that the patient/co-worker/friend/family member is a smoker themselves, If I believe the answer is yes, I may then choose to share my story. I'm always humbled by how well-received this information is with those I choose to share it with. Maybe it's because it comes from a source of genuine care and concern and absolutely no judgment. I can only pray that acceptance and understanding are what flows from my heart to theirs.

I've often wondered what other challenges health professionals have struggled with that could also help other humans? Although I personally don't suffer from an eating disorder, I know so many that do. If you have struggled with that challenge yourself could you possibly, more empathically, connect with a person who is also struggling? Maybe you've recovered from this challenge. Could you help point others in that direction because of your own battle with that disorder? Could you help that patient connect with a counselor who specializes in eating disorders? Just letting someone know they are not alone and not judged can be the first step along their road to recovery. As I previously mentioned, I truly believe nothing in life is ever wasted, not even our challenges.

How about the emotional challenges of divorce? Have you personally experienced that in your life? What about your parents or your children? I tell you, being able to support someone going through the hardships of divorce is what love really looks like to me. You can just see a deep level of understanding in someone's eyes when they've been down the road you are now walking. Whether it is you reaching out to offer support, or a patient walking alongside you in support, either way, love and understanding are exchanged. You see, sometimes our hardships help others recover from theirs. Sometimes, it's the reversal and someone else is supporting us. If you're willing to share your experience, strength and hope I believe miracles happen. There is a wonderful story that highlights my thoughts on this topic.

> There was a person who stumbled out of a bar very intoxicated, fell down into a hole and got stuck. A concerned person walked past, looked down into the hole and asked the person if they needed any money to help get them out of the hole. That didn't work. Another person came along, looked into the hole and asked if some compassionate counseling would help get them out. While that too seemed very sincere, it didn't work either. Finally, another person came along. This person saw the one stuck in the hole, climbed down into the hole and said

> to this stranger, "I can help. Will you let me?" The person asked why he thought he could help him get out when others couldn't. He replied, "I too have stumbled out of many bars intoxicated. I've fallen down many dark holes in my life. I'm healthy now and I know how to get out of this hole. I've been there before. Just take my hand and I'll show you how to climb out. We'll do it together. You're not alone"

So, what's your story? What part of your past can you be liberated from, make peace with? Don't let it hold you down from being the best person you were purposed to be. We live in a world today that offers wonderful services, many support groups and others who have walked down the road you are on. Find a way to free yourself from your past. Learn from everything and don't hesitate to share that learning with others. You don't have to confess your past with every person or patient you encounter but you will need to release the shame and guilt of the situation. Don't let your past hold you back. There is so much freedom and compassion waiting for you and those you serve. You are not alone!

Reflection:

Take a tender moment to honestly reflect on any strongholds that are holding you captive. If you feel safe, consider noting that information. Once you've identified your concerns why not write a letter to yourself that would include self-love and understanding for the baggage you've been carrying. Look to see if there is a support group, a friend, counselor, doctor and/or religious confidant that you could confide in. You don't have to carry this weight on your own. There is help out there. You are not alone and you are worth it!

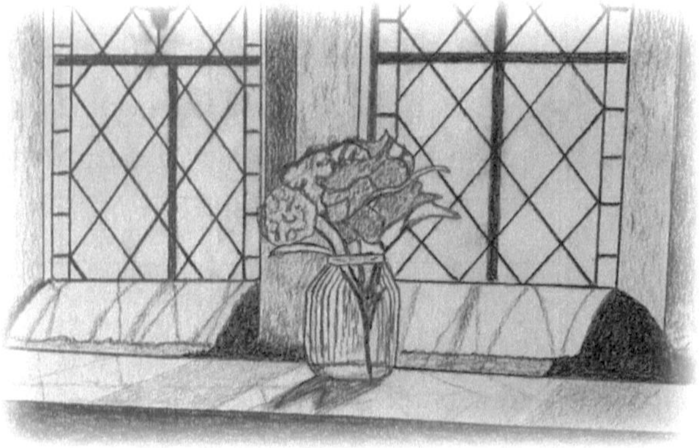

Take the Hospitality Challenge!

I cannot emphasize enough how much the simple gesture of hospitality means in the healthcare profession or, in my opinion, life! Hospitality is "the quality or disposition of receiving and treating guests and strangers in a warm, friendly, generous way." Warm. Friendly. Generous. Right from the gate, make that your priority. Employ or work with staff who are dripping with kindness. Special souls that can easily make eye contact with every person walking through your doors and greet them with a genuine smile. The type of person who can keep their cool when things are getting chaotic. A person who can be on a phone call and still look up to smile at a patient coming their way. Staff members who are eager to offer your patients assistance in meeting their needs whether there are insurance questions, financial concerns, appointment inquiries or any number of questions one might have. A person who has an approachable demeanor rather than a defensive personality. A hospitality hero.

If you really want your office to shine in this area, I strongly encourage you to begin by seeking out and then supporting your front desk staff in the hospitality challenge. They are your hospitality front-line workers. Think about some of their challenges though. It is incredibly difficult to maintain a welcoming posture when a person is interrupted all day long. Just think about that for a moment. I've often wondered, on average, how many times a day do front desk staff members get interrupted? I can't even imagine! As a kindness to that effort, minimize your interruptions when possible. Remember that it is usually your front desk team that begins the relationship with each patient and usually completes that appointment relationship too. It can become a beautiful dance, whether the pace is at jitterbug or waltz. Just keep dancing. It is just critical that you find staff to fit that special niche and then commit to wrapping your support around them in turn.

Let's also remember how important hospitality is between co-workers as well. Trust me on this. Your patients can pick up on discourse very easily. Sadly, I believe we can all relate to entering a place of business where you instantly pick up on difficulties between team members. Work hard to build healthy relationships between team members, where respect and kindness are the norm. Help foster those relationships and protect them as well. In my opinion, healthy relationships between coworkers are priceless and can springboard into your patient's hearts as well. Hospitality happens there too.

I also believe there are so many simple acts of hospitality that have the potential to catapult your business to the next level. Evaluate your waiting room space, your patient restroom facility. Does your office provide free Wi-Fi? How about your online presence? Now, more than ever, simple postings of kindness and encouragement on social platforms can communicate how much you care about your patients. I believe projecting hospitality online is not even an option anymore. If you are not tech-savvy then find someone who is. Your online presence is absolutely critical today. Critical to every generation. My parents and in-laws are both just as comfortable looking up online reviews as their grandchildren are. I'm not suggesting you lighten up on other hospitality aspects though. Just make sure you don't overlook this virtual space of hospitality either.

How does hospitality play out in your outdoor space? What about your parking lot? Is your parking lot missing pieces of asphalt or is it safe to navigate? During the

Covid 19 Pandemic, the parking lot became known as the "new" waiting room for many businesses. Can you freshen that outdoor space up with flowers? New landscaping? How about installing a simple bike rack for those that cycle for transportation? How effective is your outdoor lighting? You don't need a large space to work any of those items in, you just need a hospitable heart to create the space. If building a warm inviting atmosphere is not your talent then ask for help. This is just too critical to be left unattended. I am hoping some of the ideas I have just shared will spark something you can apply to your outdoor atmosphere. Spaces you can personalize to fit the needs of your business, team members and patients.

So let's head back inside our healthcare buildings again. I would also encourage your back-office staff to brainstorm some simple actions they could take to help patients feel more welcomed and secure once they arrive. Make sure each patient is called back with a genuine smile, even if it's behind a protective mask and face shield. Hold open all doors for them. Make sure your posture and tone of voice show respect and kindness for every patient you serve, even those arriving late or with negative attitudes. You never know what someone else is going through. You never know what battles they are facing or what loads they are carrying. Fight off the instinct to judge anyone. Just accept your patient with a kind heart and do your best. Remember, your attitude can set the tone for the time you have scheduled with your patient. Commit to generous hospitality. You can never go wrong.

You may also find it beneficial to look around your space from the view of a patient. Sit in your patient's chair. Is it comfortable? If not, consider purchasing small memory foam pillows to support your patient's neck and/or lower back. It might take you a few extra moments to unbag and re-bag these pillows but what an act of kindness and comfort for your patients. What about your wall space? Does it need freshening up? Take some time to make those choices as well. How about an informative yet decorative bulletin board? There is so much you can do with scrapbook paper, corkboard and computer ink to help educate and inform your patients. You may also want to consider having a comfortable chair in your operatory for additional family members, if allowed, to sit in while they wait. This may sound trite, but it can set a very positive tone of hospitality.

I have also found the simple gesture of letter writing to be received well by others too. In the past, I have purchased simple postcards and then chosen at least one patient per day to send a note of encouragement to. My words are always simple, yet very heartfelt. "I enjoyed spending time with you today and sharing a smile." As simple as that, I would handwrite that message and drop it in the mailbox on my way home from work. I was careful not to share any personal information, just words of kindness and encouragement. I must admit that children and the elderly shared the loveliest responses to receiving those postcards.

I also believe included with this hospitality challenge is the adaption to include patients with all expressions of abilities. Accessibility language and actions need to be a part of your healthcare practice and I believe your personal life as well. What good is a warm and welcoming staff and atmosphere if someone with a disability cannot manage the office stairs or even open a heavy door? I discovered this difficulty after a boating accident I encountered that resulted in surgical repair of my left leg. During my healing process, I needed to utilize crutches. This time in my life truly opened my eyes to what others with lifelong disabilities encounter on a day-to-day basis. Here are just a few things I learned from this life experience that can easily be applied to any healthcare office:

> Don't just meet accessibility codes. Exceed them. Be generous with wheelchair accommodations! Make sure your restrooms are suited for all abilities. Be quick to help open a door for someone. Make a phone call for transportation assistance all with a polite, not arrogant or pity-filled, attitude.
>
> Have staff take the worst parking spaces available. Think of all your patients. Not just those with disabilities. New moms with baby carriers

that contain precious cargo will greatly appreciate parking near the office door.

If you live in a climate that produces ice and snow, stay on top of those issues. As tricky as it is for someone with typical movement abilities to manage snow and ice, those issues are magnified for the elderly and/or those with disabilities. Be aware and vigilant with your outdoor safety issues.

Thankfully, many accessibility issues today have been resolved and improved upon greatly. Just check things out every so often to make sure you have a barrier-free and welcoming environment. Many cities today have local Disability Networks that are willing to come in and walk through your healthcare office to offer suggestions. I believe we need to be aware of building codes that affect the structures of our offices but what about the simple things such as signage for the hearing impaired? Placement of rugs that may impede the use of a cane or wheelchair? Whatever modifications you make, try and remember, people with disabilities are people first. Even the language you use can set a tone of hospitality by remembering to use everyone's name first before you state their unique ability. For example, my name is Judy and I

> wear glasses. Not, I'm a person with a vision challenge named Judy. Know and remember someone's name. It's a small difference but can set a completely different tone of respect and hospitality.

So, take the hospitality challenge and walk through your building inside and out. I encourage you to address all challenges that may be affecting the ability to welcome others into your space. What message does your team send during the day to your patients and even co-workers? Think about it. Is your heart filled with good, loving thoughts when you begin your workday or are anger and frustration spilling out of you? This is not always easy to address but look for small simple ways to offer someone who is struggling the gift of acceptance and welcome. I believe hospitality is both seen and felt. It begins at the very entrance of your healthcare facility and must be woven into your hearts as well.

Reflection:

Take a moment to capture what you believe your office does well regarding hospitality. What steps do you already do that set you apart? Be honest. Are there areas that you could improve upon? Make note of those and be willing to work with your team to help enhance your hospitality. Remember, you, and everyone else, are worth it!

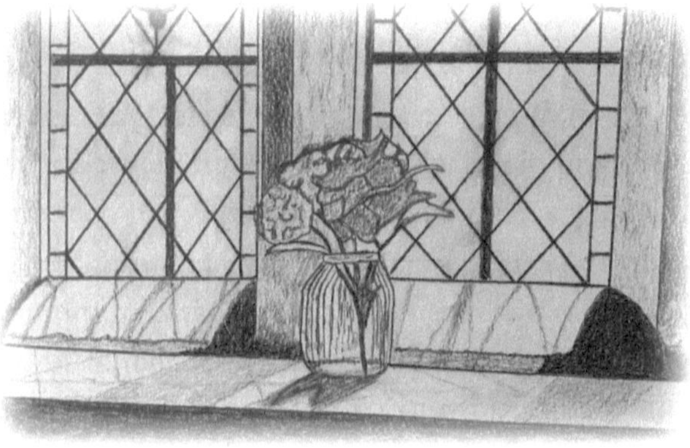

Staying In Your Moment

I can still vividly recall this moment in time like it was yesterday. Every detail still remains frozen in my mind and heart. And you know what? I don't want those precious memories to melt away either. Friend, I'd like you to meet my hero. The child who changed my life forever.

Picture this. You enter the waiting room to call back a 10-year-old child. You've worked with this joy-filled young person and his family for a few years and have developed a wonderful relationship with them. As his Mom is reviewing the medical history form you begin making eye contact with the young child. Trying to elicit a smile from his sweet face you immediately notice that he is shyly hiding under a ball cap. His skin is pale, his hair appears very wispy, there is no smile on his face today, yet his beautiful eyes seem to pierce your soul. Something just doesn't seem right though. And when my intuition flag goes off, so do my fear responses. Welcome rapid heart rate and shallow breathing as they begin their rollercoaster climb up.

My next glance allowed me to see the health updates on his medical history that included the words "cancer, chemotherapy." Well, if you're anything like me, whatever grace and strength you have at those moments must go into automatic to keep from puddling onto the waiting room floor. Even typing these words today, reliving that moment in my mind, still hurts my heart. I have a feeling, everyone reading this can also connect to that type of emotional pain. It runs deep. It seems to affect every system in our human bodies when another soul, especially a child, is suffering.

But somehow, despite my emotional pain, I needed to tap into a source greater than myself to move with this child and his mother back to my operatory room. The strength, my friend, that in my opinion, would need to be more than just my own. Truthfully, my only real memories of walking down that hallway were of shaky legs and a very dry mouth. But as I just shared, I also believe that a Higher Power fueled the strength and compassion I needed to tap into at that precious moment in time.

Strength and compassion that I never thought possible on my own but thankfully showed up in my soul.

I have no doubt each one of us has already walked down one or more of those life-changing hallways. We've chosen to go shoulder to shoulder, heart to heart, alongside someone suffering with the challenges of chronic illnesses. Maybe we've had to carry the burden ourselves of chronic illness. If it hasn't happened yet in your lifetime, it will. It is a part of life as we know it. What I'd like to share with you is what my hero taught me in a matter of seconds! So hold onto your hat and your heart!

After entering my operatory room, my hero proceeded to sit in the patient's chair while his Mom took a corner seat nearby. Mom was amazing! Absolute beauty and strength inside one tiny body. She was just happily expressing to me that the entire family was preparing to leave for Disney World thanks to the Make a Wish organization[8]. My hero was still extremely quiet but I thought to myself, as I was reclining his patient chair back, that perhaps Disney World would be a fun and safe conversation to have with him. So, I looked into my hero's eyes and asked him excitedly," So where exactly are you going?" He looked back up at me, somewhat confused, and simply answered, "backward?"

Backward. How profound. My hero taught me right then and there to stay in the moment. Stay right in the

[8] http://www.wish.org/ Make a Wish National Foundation

moment. I have no business projecting my worries or fears of the future onto anyone. I have no business dragging someone back into their past either. Whether I am treating a patient with incipient tooth decay or leukemia, my job is to stay right then and there with my patient. Stay right in their moment. It really is that simple. Talk or listen to your patient but stay in their moment, whatever that looks like to them. My hero knew that and taught me well. He wasn't leaving for Florida for 7 whole days but he was moving backward in my chair right at the moment.

I challenge you to stay in the moment with each patient you serve. Whether you are present to struggles or celebrations, stay in the moment. Don't miss any of it, it's where life really happens. I suspect most of our heroes' have learned to stay in their moments. Moments filled with bravery, compassion and love. It's where heroes like my friend lived. Thanks for teaching me this sweet life lesson friend. Thanks for coming into my life and into my heart, forever.

Reflection:

Take a moment to recognize the heroes in your life that have blessed you. Write down their names. Honor their memory. Honor your relationship with them. If tears need to flow, let them. If smiles grow, allow that to happen too. However, your body needs to process your hero's gifts, honor that, because you're worth it and so is their memory.

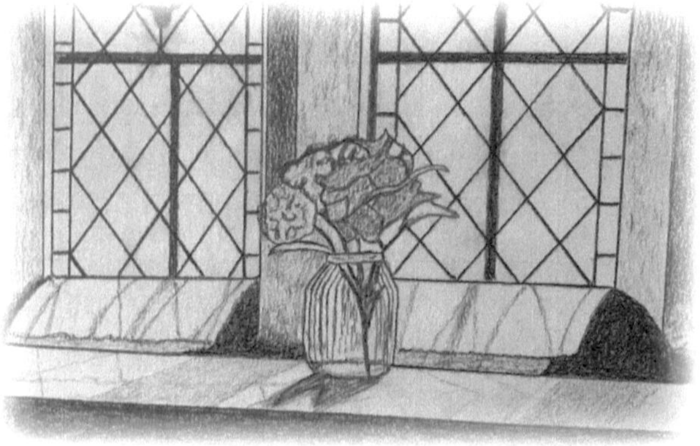

Soft Heart. Strong Back.

Years ago, when I began to practice yoga (emphasis on the word practice) I would hear the phrase "soft heart, strong back" over and over again. In some ways, those two phrases didn't seem to marry well with me. But, really think about it. Soft heart, strong back. Does it ring any bells when you think of practicing dentistry or other health professions? Could there be a hidden connection there for us? For me there is. Just the act of holding myself in a healthy posture alignment during a dental procedure requires a strong reliance on my back muscles. In every position I am in, every patient I serve, I also attempt to have my heart soft and open. I truly believe that to work in the health profession these two worlds must merge. How beautiful it is when they do.

I am so blessed to personally experience, on a daily basis, the convergence of these two worlds. Softness and strength. When a patient or even coworker presents themselves with physical, mental and/or emotional challenges, trust me, harnessing softness and strength will help you move through your day more easily. It's these moments that I attempt to tap into my breath though, in order to activate both strength and softness. To keep feelings of defensiveness and frustration at bay. Unfortunately, my default behaviors can still trip me up, sinking me into despair and/or discouragement. I've learned though, from the beautiful expression of yoga, that focusing on my breath can bring about a sense of calm. This inner peace then seems to make space for my brain to stay online as well as my heart to remain engaged. I no longer need to "tune someone out" in order to survive a difficult appointment or coworker interaction. I can stay tuned into my breath, remain present to the situation and strong enough to move with grace through it. Do I do this perfectly? Not even close! But I love the challenge and I wholeheartedly believe it is worth it.

One of the simplest examples I can offer you when a strong back and soft heart collide can happen at the beginning of your day. Back story. I have purposed to begin my day well in advance of seeing my first patient.

While I am home, I choose to meditate and eat a balanced breakfast before I leave for the office. When I arrive, I go through my patient charts, hone all instruments, review the daily schedule and attend a staff huddle. I've got my game face on. I am ready to go and serve everyone coming through my operatory door. Well, it doesn't happen often, but when my first patient of the day arrives late, in the past it used to create enormous tension in my whole body. I projected that I would be running behind for the rest of the morning. I could almost visualize the look every subsequent patient would offer me, wondering why I was running behind.

This behavior, my friends, is not one that I am proud of. You see, on any given day, with any given patient, I personally can run behind all on my own. Why then would I project those toxic feelings onto my first patient of the day when I knew nothing of their life circumstances? Well, those behaviors and feelings all began to unravel when I started my yoga practice. Although I can't do a downward dog in my operatory, I can always bring in the calming effects of breathwork at any moment. And this, my friend, has been a game-changer. I can now stand in grace, no matter the awkwardness of the situation, grounded in strength and compassion. Again, not always perfectly, but I do show up with that intention every day.

So why the connection between yoga and the health profession? I think it's because of the unexpected blessings yoga has brought to my life. It has made me realize that I do present myself to my patients with a soft heart. A heart willing to bend, to absorb, to hold gently the person I am working with. Yet, it is with the strength of my back that holds me upright, that provides me the endurance to be more physically present to the one I am serving. And the gel that holds all this together for me is my breathwork. Deeply breathing in and purposely exhaling out. Feeling the movement of air through my nostrils. Being aware of the air movement in my chest and abdomen is so simple yet so effective. I've heard it said that one cannot fall back to the past or project into the future when they are focused on their present breath. This simple act forces the mind and body to stay in the present moment. To stay in the treasured space where you can choose calm and clarity over frustration. In that space your brain can stay online helping you to see clearly, helping you to choose your words and actions wisely.

Do I think yoga is the only way to achieve this balance of life? Absolutely not. We are all wired for different physical and emotional needs. I have had co-workers who thrive on running marathons coupled with regular massage therapy. These humans are amazing, beautiful, strong and serene. Their way just isn't my way. Nor should it be. Question is, what is your way? How can you achieve the physical and emotional balance needed to be truly present to the one you are serving while still becoming your personal best? Whatever you do, just find a way to keep your heart in the lead. Trust me, you won't regret it.

Reflection:

Spend some time experimenting with what actions most bring you peace and calm. Are you most calm after you work out in the morning before you head to work? Are you more calm meditating before you arrive at the office? Try both and see how you feel. And don't be hard on yourself. This process may take a while. Just remember, soft heart and a strong back and you're so worth it!

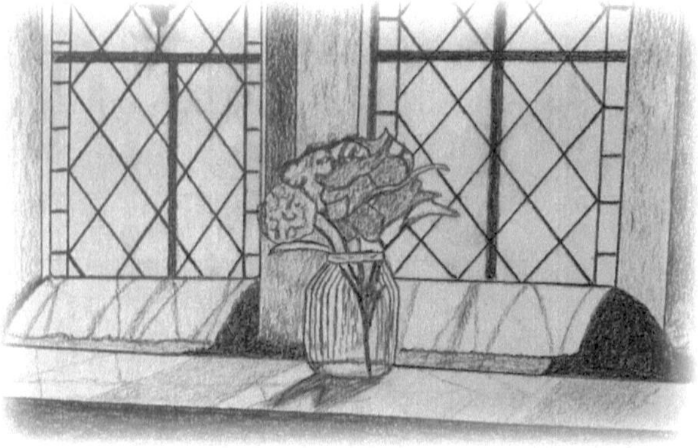

What Brand Are You?

So how does one keep their heart in the lead if they aren't familiar with the rhythm of their own heart? Think about it. How can we attempt to project softness and strength to those we serve when we can't identify what exactly gives pulse to our own heart muscle? What provides us softness? What strengthens our mind, body and soul? Ready to have some fun finding out? Let's go for it!

Picture this. You're searching for employment. You've tuned up your interviewing skills, did the appropriate background searches on prospective employers, cleaned up your online social media platforms, designated an interviewing outfit and possibly spent hours fine-tuning your resume. When all this work pays off, and it will, you are contacted to come for an interview. At this moment, there might be a few butterflies in your stomach, the rumblings of a hurricane or even possible ecstatic shouts of joy. Either way, the opportunity to sit down with a prospective employer and begin a conversation is going to happen. Whatever the underlying currents of emotions are, know you are not alone. You are enough. And you've already succeeded by just obtaining the interview. But we also know that it typically requires more than a good resume and interview suit to land a job. It's going to take connections. Multiple layers of connections. Connecting to your true self, to your profession, to your community, to the healthcare team you would like to be a part of. Believe it or not, unraveling these layers or finding ways to connect them together, is actually quite simple. Stay with me.

I'd love to share with you a process that I believe will help you begin uncovering your true self. To help you define what exactly brings rhythm to your heartbeat. To help you then project your true image onto others while seeking employment or any other facet of your life. To eventually, with confidence and joy, bring these personal discoveries into full view. So, what am I talking about? Have you ever heard of personal branding? Don't laugh, but the first time I heard the phrase "branding" my only reference point was the process of cattle identification and I'm not even connected to the ranching industry. Thankfully I didn't brush over the phrase. You see, personal branding is simply the process of self-discovery and the ability to apply what you've learned to your personal and professional lifestyle.

I must admit that I had done very little self-discovering in my life. I could tell you what each of my four children and husband liked. I could even share lots of information about siblings, parents and other family members. But for myself? What made me, me? I was lost. And so, I began my own journey of personal discovery after reading a blog post my daughter, Ashley Nelson, had written while she was in college. I can still remember digesting that information and asking myself why had I never done this before? Could this process really be that simple? Would discovering more about myself be of any professional or personal benefit? Well, I decided to dive in. Glad I did. This journey made such an impact on me that my daughter and I developed a Continuing Education program on this topic. We were able to share our personal branding passions with dental hygiene students as well as other dental professionals. It was a blast!

So, if I haven't lost you yet, let me share a very broad view of our workshop. We began by helping each participant discover what colors, shapes and even words they responded to. We then helped each participant unravel and integrate these learnings into their resume, business cards and clothing attire. Just a side note. Even if you are not looking for a new place of employment, a person can always benefit from discovering their personal brand. Because whether you like it or not, you have a personal brand. Taking the time to discover it, fine-tune it and own it will truly set you apart. The interpersonal connections made when discovering your personal brand, I believe, are endless.

It was thrilling to see the light in our participant's eyes shine a little brighter when they uncovered another layer of self-identity during our workshop. This program is so simple and has the potential to grow a deeper understanding and confidence for each participant involved. And I believe, when the confidence flows, so many wonderful things will also fall into place.

So, why not spend a little time to uncover more of you? I hope you consider this challenge and then fully embrace what you discover. There are several user-friendly online sites that can guide you through this journey. I personally love learning more about the Psychology of Color. If you want a sneak-peek into that world, the following is a quick rundown of how color might play out in your life. The chart which follows contains a generalized synopsis of personality attributes that are commonly found associated with particular colors. Keep in mind the chart is just a glimpse into a beautiful study of color. You can always go deeper. Believe me, it will be a joyful journey you won't regret.

- **Red** – strength, passion, energy, bold
- **Blue** – Intelligence, trust, efficiency, serenity
- **Yellow** – Optimism, confidence, friendly, creative
- **Green** – Harmony, economical, energy, ecofriendly
- **Orange** – Security, passion, energetic, warmth
- **Pink** – Tranquility, love, adventurous, emotional
- **Black** – Sophistication, security, efficiency, daring

Any guesses what my favorite color is? Even if you don't know me, you might be able to rule a few colors out just by reading my writing. My favorite color has been and probably always will be green. Do I identify with only green color attributes though? Is that my entire brand? Absolutely not. I move very gently in and out of the color palate. I just seem to always find myself bringing shades of green back into my life as my dominant color choice.

I wonder what your favorite color is and what that might say about you. I wonder what brings rhythm to your heartbeat. Whatever that answer is, I don't think we can deny that some shades of color will stand out to us at different times in our lives. We are very fluid creatures who are hopefully learning and growing every day. So, why not embrace what brings you joy today. Look for the blessings in all you do and the world will smile back at you. Take the time to discover your brand. To deepen connections in your life. Own your brand! Know the cadence of your heart because you are so worth it!

Reflection:

Find some time to yourself in the near future. Begin by checking out the Psychology of Color resources and see where this journey takes you. Look around you. Look within you. See what makes you, you. And then own it because you are so worth it!

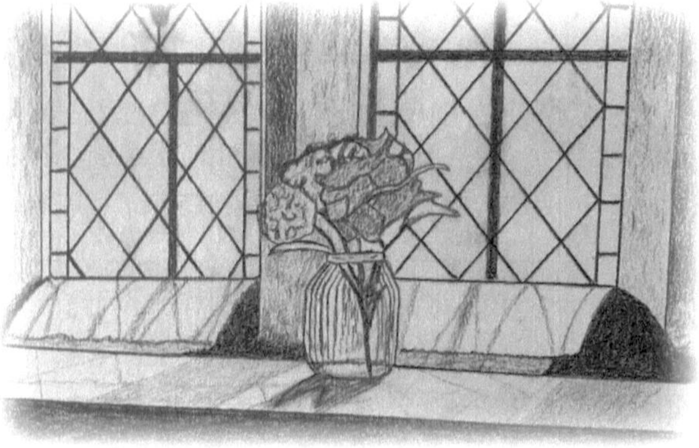

Don't Judge a Book by Her Cover

I know. It's an old axiom we've all heard countless times. One must never judge a book by its cover. If you looked closely enough, I titled this chapter and used the pronoun "she" instead of "it." Yes, there is a reason for that. One, however, I am not especially proud of.

It's been over 40 years since I graduated from a dental hygiene program and I am sure I have forgotten many educational and clinical details that were taught to me by my brilliant professors. For some reason, the name "Esther Wilkens" has never been forgotten by me, though. Sadly,

I never developed a sense of respect while I was a student for this amazing woman when reading her book *Clinical Practice of the Dental Hygienist.* Instead, I looked at this gift with a fearful attitude while studying for tests, and ultimately, my National Board Exam. For some twisted reason, I thought this beautiful and brilliant woman had it out for me. I'd never met Esther, but I still had it in my head she was trying to sabotage my dental hygiene success by developing such a brilliant handbook of dental hygiene for me to memorize. What I have since come to realize is that all along, Esther Wilkens had her heart and soul behind my career success. It was I who tainted it with my fear of failure.

So, how did I find myself tangled up in judgment and fear instead of acceptance and freedom? It's a long story and one too convoluted to get into right now. Needless to say, today I intentionally choose not to live in fear or judgment. Today I choose not to judge a book by its cover. Now I have a clearer view of life's library right before my eyes. Today I work very hard to not judge anything or anyone by their cover. I take it off the shelf. I unwrap it. I look, I listen. I discuss it with a trusted friend or colleague if necessary. I am even known to research the topic to increase my understanding. This doesn't mean I always agree with the issue. I just no longer prematurely cast judgment on a topic or person.

If you too are a part of the healthcare profession, I believe it is critical to leave fear and judgment out of our educational experience, our workplace and our lives. The relationships we will forge will be built on genuineness and not a mountain of fear. We'll still make mistakes but will have the skills to learn from them and not to be paralyzed by them. I invite you to challenge yourself to remain open-minded and not judgeful. If you have errors from your past you need to deal with, I encourage you to make amends. Accept that you were doing the best you could at the time but want to live free from the shackles of those challenges. For me, making amends came in the form of an email I composed to Esther many years ago. Although I never heard back from her, I was copied that it was forwarded to her home email address. With an open heart, I share with you the following:

Message of thanks from a 1981 Kellogg Community College Graduate

Dear Ms. Wilkins,

This note of thanks should never have waited 31 years to be sent. Your book, *Clinical Practice of the Dental Hygienist* was my lifeline while in hygiene school and is still a mainstay for me today.

As I look back on my dental hygiene career, I am aware of the many blessings I have received. It remains an honor for me to work in this career field. I do regret never having acknowledged your brilliance though. I spent most of my time as a student being fearful and intimidated of your published work. I hope today you can receive my VERY overdue and genuine note of thanks.

I recently read that you were recovering from a health situation this past June. I pray you have recovered and continue to feel energized. I and many other hygienists still need you! Because of you (and many others) I left my fears behind and began submitting articles for consideration to be published in the *RDH* magazine. I am happy to report that several articles were published (with the help of editor Mark Hartley and staff.) You were my inspiration!

So, in closing, I wish you a beautiful day and the chance to share your smile with another. Thank you for giving me the voice and privilege to work in such an amazing profession!

God bless you always,
Judith Stein RDH
Kellogg Community College, 1981

This dear woman never responded to my email but in my heart of hearts, I pray she felt my admiration and respect. Esther passed away four years after I sent this email. She was blessed to have lived 100 years on this earth and remains a legacy in the dental hygiene profession. With great respect and thankfulness, I share an excerpt from her online obituary.

Esther M. Wilkins Gallagher, RDH, DMD, 100, formerly of Tyngsborough, Massachusetts, died Monday, December 12th at Laurel Place of Fairview Healthcare in Hudson, New Hampshire. She was the beloved wife of the late James B. Gallagher, Jr., DMD. Esther was also the sister of the late Ruth Wilkins Colby. Dr. Wilkins is survived by a niece Elisabeth C. Tyrol of Pelham, NH; and many grandnieces, grandnephews, great-grandnieces and great-grandnephews.

Born in Chelmsford, Massachusetts, December 9, 1916, the daughter of the late Ernest and the late Edith (Packard) Wilkins, she attended Tyngsboro schools and was a graduate of Lowell High School in the Class of 1934. Eager to further her education, she then went on to graduate from Simmons College in Boston with a Bachelor of Science degree in 1938. She then continued on to graduate from Forsyth School of Dental Hygiene in 1939 and then earn a Doctor of Dental Medicine degree from Tufts School of Dental Medicine in 1949. In 1966 she earned a certificate in periodontology from Tufts as well.

She was a Dental Educator and Professor Emeritus at Tufts School of Dental Medicine. Dr. Wilkins was known to have dedicated her life to her work. She traveled extensively and internationally mentoring and lecturing. She wrote and had published "Clinical Practice of the Dental Hygienist" which was printed in 12 editions. It is known as the bible and roadmap to Dental Hygienists all over the world and was translated into six different languages.

Reflection:

I believe that making amends is a priceless gift you can share with another and also receive yourself. Sometimes it requires a simple, yet brave apology. Sometimes it's more complicated and you may need to seek counsel for direction. Whatever needs to happen, know you are not alone. Talk things over with a trusted friend and begin your road to living free from your past and help someone else move forward in theirs because you are worth it!

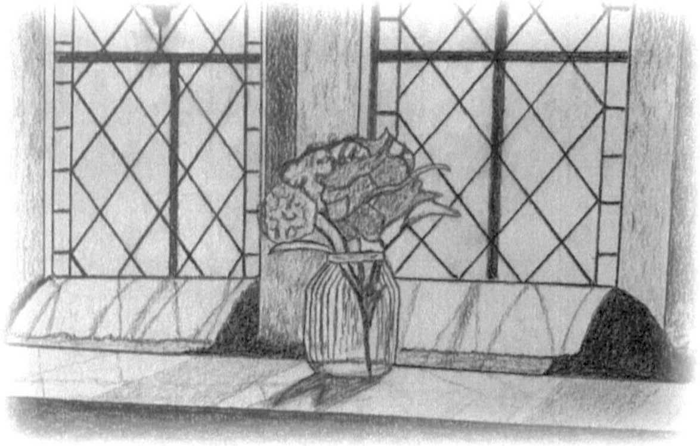

Two Sides of the Same Coin

Interested in living in the judgment-free zone? Curious how to get there? Wondering how to navigate life's obstacles, those dreaded orange cones of road construction along the journey? Well, buckle up. I'd like to personally invite you to begin cultivating an ability to view different perspectives of a person or circumstance in order for you to arrive at that destination. To see both sides of the same coin. Both sides of the same dilemma. To continue living non-judgmentally and be willing to put the work into growing that critical life skill. Could you just imagine our world if we all put those beliefs into practice?

If we chose to leave judgment behind us at every threshold we entered in order to view life more openly? I'd like to say I have always lived judgment-free but that wouldn't be the truth. Thankfully though, today I am more aware when my thinking becomes distorted and I begin down the judgment road. Today, I am personally and professionally committed to viewing every side of a coin without the lens of judgment clouding over my view. All I can say is what took me so long!

So how exactly has this life skill played out in my life? For starters, it's helped me realize that although we may not all line up with similar viewpoints, we are all entitled to our opinions. I must remind myself often, that in general, there are at least two sides to every topic and I must attempt to remain in an empathetic, neutral zone of awareness as often as possible. It's not enough for me to will judgment away from my thought process though. Instead, I have found replacing it with empathy and understanding has become a very helpful strategy. Living this way helps keep frustration and clouded judgment from seeping into my thoughts and behaviors. It's not easy, but living this way is so worth it.

Intentionally living more empathetically has been a huge blessing to me especially when controversial topics are brought up. Topics such as national elections, pandemic responses and many others which carry a high risk of separating you from your patient and or coworker. As healthcare professionals, we must caution ourselves from bringing certain personal opinions to work, some sensitive topics have the grave potential to taint working relationships and possibly alter the health effect we hope to accomplish with our patients. Even with our best intentions, I'm afraid the risk of these controversies seeping into our working environment is very high. Even if you don't initiate the conversation, believe me, it will happen. When it does, you can try to remain neutral if possible. Plug into empathy and understanding if you can. I must confess though. I have a few hot topics that I cannot tolerate. My line in the sand so to speak. I'm guessing you have a few unbendable opinions you hold as well. When and if those conversations come up, I try to calmly address them. It is always my hope to plant seeds of understanding and not shame even if I disagree with someone's opinion. I have to remind myself that everyone is doing their best, including me.

Let's take this show on the road if you don't mind. See how we can plug it into life. Before I begin down this road though, I'd like to thank all those judgment-free souls that have shown me, have mentored me, how to live life more fully. Thank you for not shaming me when I projected judgment when I should have been spilling out empathy and understanding. You too are heroes in my world. You have filled the world with hope, understanding and peace.

All right, let's venture forth. For me, a clear example of viewing both sides of the same coin happens when I substitute in another work setting. Whatever healthcare modality you are connected to, the possibility to substitute usually exists. Although I have primarily worked from a home base dental environment, where the familiar routines and faces reside, I have also had the honor of working as a substitute hygienist in several dental offices throughout my career. I have certainly learned many valuable lessons during that time. Lessons I may not have experienced had I not ventured away from my home base. Although I may not feel comfortable taking such risks, I believe there will always be a blessing connected to that action. As I mentioned, there are always two sides to the same coin and substituting can offer you a front-row seat to that view.

What about the times when a coworker, friend or family member has a different opinion than you on a topic? Suppose you don't agree with their suggestions or their way of handling a situation? This, my friend, used to charge my emotions with feelings of intense dread. If I disagreed with their suggestions, how could I address the issue without severing the relationship? What if I agreed, just to keep the peace, but deep down I didn't really agree? Can you relate? Well, it wasn't until I began to actively leave judgment out of my thought process and intentionally brought empathy in, did I finally experience the freedom to view every side of every coin. If I agreed, that's easy. If their opinion differed from mine though, I try to actively listen more. If I still didn't agree or there is still conflict at the end of the discussion I will simply state,

"Although I don't agree with your suggestion, you might be right." I don't state they are right, I declared they might be right. Phrasing my thoughts this way leaves room for continued conversation from both parties. Continued discovery. Continued growth. And what a game-changer. I no longer dread confrontation because I don't look at it that way anymore. Instead, I keep my mind open and curious. And I love living this way.

So don't be surprised to discover many hidden blessings and treasures on both sides of every coin you uncover. Whether it is learning to live free of judgment or keeping an open mind. Whatever side of the coin you find yourself on, I promise you there will be magic waiting for you.

Reflection:

Get honest. Do some inner work to discover where and if you harbor judgment that is impacting your personal and work relationships. Be willing to identify those areas and see if you can counteract that action with empathetic understanding. It may be subtle at first but commit to growing this attribute. Not only will you enjoy the fruits of this skill but the world around you will also reap a multitude of blessings. Go for it, because you are worth it!

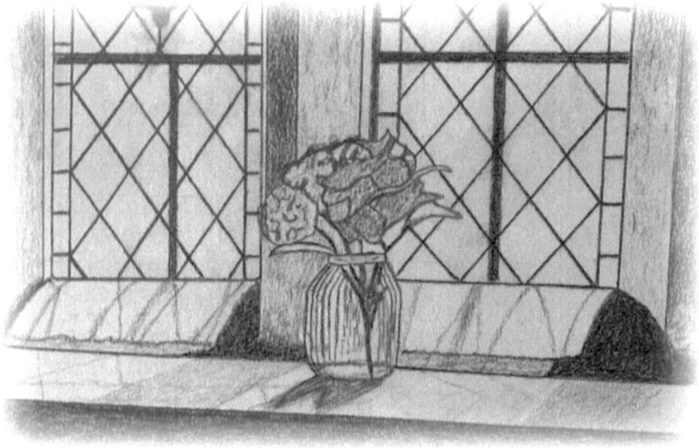

I Was Rescued

A bird is safe in its nest — but that is not what its wings are made for.

Amit Ray

Truth. Burnout can happen, even to the best of us. Moving through a global pandemic can certainly acerbate the effects of burnout, both at a personal and professional level. Anyone alive in 2020, during the Covid 19 global pandemic, can relate to the challenges of burnout. Essential workers by the thousands were stretched physically, mentally and emotionally for months as we waged war against an invisible virus. When dental offices were allowed to open, it was all hands-on deck as many struggled to catch back up. Unfortunately, burnout took the careers of many healthcare professionals too early. As many of us fought to survive our own stress storms, to manage the effects of our own personal burnout, we weren't able to support our fellow practitioners at times. Something I deeply regret. Many retired early. Many opted to find other careers. In hindsight, I wish I could have reached out to help prevent this from happening to others. Thankfully, I had had my own professional "awakening" years ago. As strange as it is for me to be thankful for that past experience, it had forced me to build a "burnout resistance strategy" routine that helped save me from the career casualties of 2020. Let me explain.

For me, I was about 15 years into my profession before burnout hit me. As I look back, it wasn't just my career that was burning out. My personal life was pretty exhausting too. I was juggling a career and a family with four children. At work, I seemed to be more focused on what stressed me out rather than what was working. When I was home, I looked pretty ragged most days too. It wasn't all horrible, I just chose to focus on the challenges instead of the blessings. Yes, I was doing my best, I was just very tired and overwhelmed.

So, what rescued me from the abyss of burn-out and exhaustion? Exercise, meditation and the *RDH* magazine. I'm serious. No, this isn't a plug for the *RDH* magazine, it's just what really helped me get back in the game. Those three elements seem to address the physical, mental and spiritual parts of my being that were struggling. You know, they say you generally get out of life what you give to it. Well, I had gotten pretty off-balance and definitely needed some recalibrating. So, little by little, as I read different articles, began a yoga practice, took a Mindfulness class, I started to awaken. Mind you, I didn't start all three things at once. It was gradual, over several years, but it was worth the effort and sustains me to this day. It began to reopen doors of learning for me, of physical and mental health as well.

I must also share that another key element to surviving personal and professional burnout for me is staying connected to a social group. Whether it is your home family, a circle of friends or your work family. It is a tremendous help to have "people" that check in with you. People that are willing to make sure you're doing ok. People you can check in on as well. For some reason, these simple heartfelt connections always remind me of a circle. I can almost visualize beautiful circles of friendship and love where connection flows around and around and around. A circle that holds and supports each member. A circle that can widen to include others at any time. A simple circle of connection to help counteract both personal and professional burnout.

So, no matter what your circle looks like today, I'd be honored to become a part of yours. If you're struggling with the effects of burnout, please know you are not alone. Maybe you could just do one thing today that would help strengthen your circle. Build some resistance to burnout. Try yoga. Go on a nature walk. Look into a meditation app. Call or text a friend. Plug into some good music. Share a hug with someone. Cut back on unnecessary commitments if possible. Whatever you feel called to do, please know and trust that I believe in you.

If the space you currently occupy is more settled, I rejoice with you! Consider sharing that joy with others though. Sometimes it just takes a subtle change of the wind to shift a person's perspective. You could be that breeze that whispers comfort into another's soul. Sometimes it takes just one person to pull another out of a burnout cycle. Sometimes that's not the case but it sure can't hurt to be available for that purpose. Right now, more than ever, our world needs a collision of circles to pull us all through. I for one will rejoice, and not complain, in a traffic jam of circles.

Reflection:

What element of your life do you need rescuing from? Are you struggling with physical, mental or emotional challenges? Maybe all three? Please remember you are not alone and maybe, just for today, you could explore an activity that brings you joy and peace. If your body and soul need to rest more, please choose rest. Whatever you need to do, go for it. And never forget, you are so worth it!

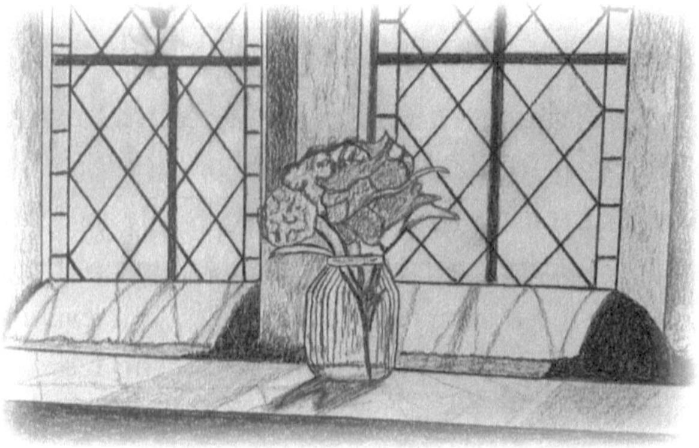

There Is No Right or Wrong Time. Just Start!

The words of Simon Sinek are timeless. "There is no right or wrong time. Just start. Better now than later and better late than never." Whether you are trying to pull yourself out of a stress cycle, stuck in the middle of a procrastination puddle or you find yourself secured in a circle of health, I believe the essence of this phrase is spot on.

If I'm being truly honest though, there is still a part of me that is silently wondering if putting this phrase into action could really be that easy. Can I really start over at any time? I've previously shared how I work through a schedule derailment and how those actions have really helped me in other areas of my life. What I have also discovered is that I still struggle with issues of control. My brain knows I can only control myself and my reactions to life, it's just there are still moments of control frustration that trip me up. Moments that creep into my soul. Issues that have the ability to set up a perfect stress storm in my life. Again, a simple example for many of us has been moving through the Coronavirus global pandemic. Prior to March 2020, my schedule was packed full of patients, whom I longed to serve. I then found myself, due to the Covid 19 pandemic crisis, at home, sewing fabric masks and, wondering if I will ever return to my beloved profession. How, and can we, really "just start over?"

Thankfully, most health professionals have been able to return to work, to our beloved careers. It's not a time in history I want to visit again but I'm so grateful for the efforts my leadership provided to me. Thanks to technology we were still able to virtually meet in order to brainstorm ways to open back up. Ways to start over again. We now have new ways of contacting patients, new ways of isolating operatory rooms, new methods of managing aerosols, and a new protocol that protects ourselves and our patients. But like the song, "make new friends but keep the old, one is silver and the other is gold," I believe we'll find treasure in both categories. In order to blend the old with the new, we needed a spirit of wisdom, flexibility, teamwork and creativity that guided us through that unprecedented time in history.

I also encourage you to never forget, no matter how many times you need to start over, that we all stand on the shoulders of those who have gone before us. I hope you remain grateful for the wonderful foundations others have left for you. Some bases were solid rock. Others show more weathering and structural challenges. If you look closely enough, I believe you'll find learning in either foundation. All we need to do is remain united, connected and committed to serving our patients with a spirit of compassion and professional excellence. Does it look different today? Yes. Do we still serve with an attitude of excellence? Absolutely yes. Will there be new mental and physical adjustments needed to help us all "start over?" Right now, I will share my thoughts with you in a spirit of hope. Hope that my thoughts will be relevant to you. If not, maybe there will be pearls you can pluck out that will still be a blessing.

So let's dig a little deeper into this topic and apply Simon's wisdom to a typical experience most of us deal with daily. Anyone struggle with the element of time management at home or at work? Can anyone else relate to the collapsing of your schedule only 30 minutes into your day? Please tell me I'm not alone. Thankfully, Simon Sinek put out some simple words of encouragement on how to start over. "There is no right or wrong time. Just start over.

Better now than later and better late than never." I love it! Take a deep breath and just start over.

Let's stay brave and explore another aspect of starting over. What if the circumstances that encouraged you to start over were the result of emotional challenges? For example, someone treats you rudely at work. You have a negative confrontation with a family member or friend. Either scenario can make it very difficult to just start over. For me, those moments always seem to leave a little emotional residue on my heart while I'm trying to "start over." And what do I do with that residue? I begin simply by trying to understand where the other person is coming from. What emotional residue do they have on their soul? What is driving their behavior? Is it fear? Loss of control? Are there painful memories of past experiences seeping into our shared space?

If I can harness some understanding, I can sometimes begin to move through the situation differently. I can more easily start over and possibly help heal the interaction. This is when a gentle transfer of understanding flows back into my heart. For me, this is when the healing begins to happen, allowing me to really "start over." If I can dig even a little deeper into my well of compassion, sometimes, by the end of the interaction, the situation has significantly turned around. When that happens, it's just a beautiful moment for both patient and practitioner.

Side note. If any of these interactions occurred in your work environment, I strongly encourage you to document the situation. This action may sound trite but trust me on this. You will never regret having made notes of the interaction. It will allow you, or the next practitioner, a chance to possibly prepare differently. Your notes will also allow you to determine if there are patterns of behavior. This could shed a tremendous amount of light on the situation. This information could ultimately help you to understand that it was never about you. Sadly, the negative baggage this person was throwing at you, was about their brokenness. These encounters are still very hard to move away from. Still very painful to shake off.

I also strongly urge you not to isolate yourself when dealing with the challenge of starting over. Who knows, others around you may have strategies that you hadn't thought of that could positively affect the situation. I have personally found that sometimes, I just need to privately ask another trusted human to help me shake off what had just happened to me. Someone to help me reframe the situation. I remind this person that I am not judging I just need help moving forward with a clean slate. I need to be heard. I truly hope you have people in your life that are there for you too. Others who don't propagate judging and are willing to help you, "shake it off" and start over again. As Simon Sinek states, "There's no right or wrong time. Just start. Better now than later and better late than never." You truly can begin your day over at any moment. Inhale all the hope of a new beginning and then exhale all the baggage of the past. Remember, you are a work in progress.

Reflection:

Spend some time contemplating how control plays out in your life. Be brave enough to see if control is an obstacle for you to "start over." Was control a contributing player that helped cause the need to start over in the first place? Be honest and gentle with yourself. See where you need to stand firm and where you can be more flexible because you are so worth it.

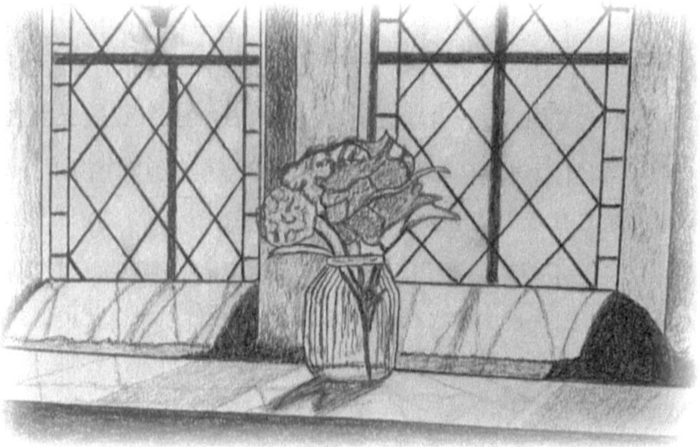

Getting Your Groove On

When you hear the word groovy, does that phrase take you back to the '70s? Can you hear the song from the Brady Bunch TV sitcom playing in your head too? I immediately see flowers painted on Volkswagen vans, fringed leather vests, silk shirts, platform shoes, hip-hugger jeans and peace signs everywhere. Well, as fun as it might sound to revisit that era, I'm hoping rather to elicit a new groove in your personal and professional psyche. A groove for organization. Yes, my friend, organization. For me though, just reading the word "organize" can evoke feelings of panic and anxiety. I've always wanted to be organized, I just never knew how or where to start. Thankfully I stumbled across the phrase "progress not perfection" a few years back. Being a closet perfectionist, I knew deep down that expectations and fears of failure were actually holding me back from becoming more organized. I longed for the freedom to unload my unhealthy baggage of perfectionism and begin working towards making progress. Deep down, I wanted every closet in my house to be Martha Stewart worthy.

Well, as luck would have it, or divine intervention, one of my patients rescued me from my organizational black hole. This lovely human shared she had recently made a career change into the world of organizational improvements. She had taken a leap of faith, left a predictable place of employment and ventured out on her own. She opened an organizational business designed to serve the needs of anyone looking to get their organizational groove on. This serendipitous meeting helped launch me out of my paralyzing space of fear and towards organizational paradise. And I was ready!

After shaking off my fear of being judged, I made an appointment to begin this journey with an organizing expert. This dear soul came over to my home (pre-pandemic), looked at the spaces that concerned me the most and helped me devise a simple plan. My organizational challenges included school papers from four children, financial paperwork and electronic data. Mind you. This paperwork wasn't thrown around my home. Oh no.

That wasn't my superpower. My superpower was the ability to expertly pile paperwork on top of chairs, tables and even the piano bench. I had become the Queen of the Pile and I was good at it. Trouble was, it took forever to locate needed information and paperwork. This method also made it hard for me to determine what should be kept and what could be recycled. Bottom line, I was an organizational mess.

So, where did I begin? Which pile did I choose to tackle first? Thankfully, my guide encouraged me to choose only one area and begin there. Well, that's what I did. I began by creating four different, easy to use, binders that would help me organize each of my children's school papers. That simple first step, that simple first action led me to create several more binders at my own pace. I collated items from appliance warranties to immunization health records. Eventually, those piles in my house were disappearing and so were the loads of frustration, fear and embarrassment I had also been carrying.

This glorious uprising at home spread into my work environment as well. It was so simple to create binders to store paperwork that I needed at work too. I can't speak for all healthcare practitioners, but many of us don't have actual office space. If you do, that is fantastic. If you don't, there is still hope. If you are like me, you may need to create one in the operatory you work out of. And that is just what I did. I created several binders that housed insurance codes, supply ordering information, water line testing paperwork, sterilization testing results and many other items I can now quickly access. Needless to say, I have continued on this path and remain committed to the simple strategies the organizational expert set me up with over 15 years ago. It has actually become addicting, in a healthy way. But don't jump off this groove train quite yet. I've got more to share.

As with so many things in my life, I stumbled across additional tools to supplement my journey towards a simpler, more organized and less cluttered life. It's like my blinders flew off and I became more aware of other organizational avenues I could explore. I came across the book, *2 Second Lean*, by Paul A Ackers.[9] This book was amazing and so very simple to put into practice. It contained many additional resources and the enthusiasm I needed to stay committed to living more organized. It helped me look at my work and personal environments in smaller segments. I would choose just one action per day to work on. Just one action. Paul suggested you begin this journey by first identifying the challenges around you and work to correct them. Not everything at once, just one action at a time. He then recommends you continuously work towards improving everything, everybody, every day. Make this process a daily habit. And finally, Paul suggests you create videos of your improvement. I choose to journal my efforts. And you guessed it, I put that information in a binder.

[9] https://paulakers.net/books/2-second-lean

Let's pause to think about this for a moment. Being willing to wake up every day and do just one thing to improve yourself and the world around you. It doesn't even have to be a grand gesture, although I would never tire of seeing that happen. For me, I just started to notice the things that frustrated me and began working towards resolving those issues. For example, a few work areas in the dental office I worked at were somewhat cluttered. I began working towards cleaning those areas up, one at a time. Since they were not my workstations alone, I also needed to collect feedback from other coworkers regarding possible changes in those workspaces. When I finally received the green light from all impacted to proceed, I chose one task a day to work on. And, believe it or not, this did not overwhelm me at all. In fact, it empowered me. I didn't need to draw attention to my actions or receive accolades for them either. It just felt good, really good.

I have also enjoyed the ideas and suggestions that author, Marie Kondo[10] has shared. She has many simple ways to organize your professional and personal life as well. I love the emphasis on the joy that Marie brings to her work. I also appreciated that I could choose my own timeline while decluttering my life. Don't hesitate to search out others that are gifted with this skill set. They are there to help you and it doesn't have to be frightening or painful.

---

[10] https://konmari.com/

Another book that has kept my organizational groove flowing is, *Stretch*, by Dr. Scott Sonenshein.[11] Oh my friends, in my humble opinion, it is a fabulous read. The book is directed towards a business audience but can absolutely be applied to any sector of society. The author encourages the reader to stretch their creativity and problem-solving skills. It is not the author's intention to stretch you in order to add more to your plate though. Not at all. The author highlights examples of different ways others have gotten stretchy in their work and home life. I have now adopted the phrase, "getting stretchy" whenever I need to brainstorm an organizational solution, a challenging life situation or find myself attempting to get stretchy doing yoga. Emphasis on the word attempting.

Another wonderful discovery along my life's journey was the realization that hidden within my coworker was an organizational pot of gold. Don't ask me how I missed it either. She, my friend, is the golden ticket to organizational heaven. My co-worker is a natural organizational expert. She just knows how to move and work in every environment she is in. She uses containers of all shapes and sizes to help organize a space. She can see spatially how items affect different workspaces. She is thoughtful when making changes that may impact my workflow too. I learned to really trust her organizational judgment. Her wisdom is a blessing to me, not a threat. If you have such

[11] https://www.scottsonenshein.com/stretch/

a gem in your home or work environment, I hope you too can recognize their gifts and let them light the way.

Living a leaner, more joy-filled life, tackling life just one action at a time is a beautiful, more sustainable way to live. Personal frustrations will happen but woven within those moments will be sparks of joy, freedom and hope. So, go for it! Find your groove and start dancing. Choose to begin living, one action, one moment at a time in a more organized manner. What do you have to lose but maybe some misery and frustrations? And trust me, you won't regret it!

Reflection:

If you need assistance in becoming more organized begin with one simple action. Consider doing an internet search for an organizational agency to help you grow in this area. Or, you could begin by doing a library search for supportive reading material. You might even discover someone you already know could help you become more organized. Whatever you do, it doesn't need to be a big step. Take the pressure off yourself right now and just take one baby step today. Who knows where that will lead you? And remember, you are worth it!

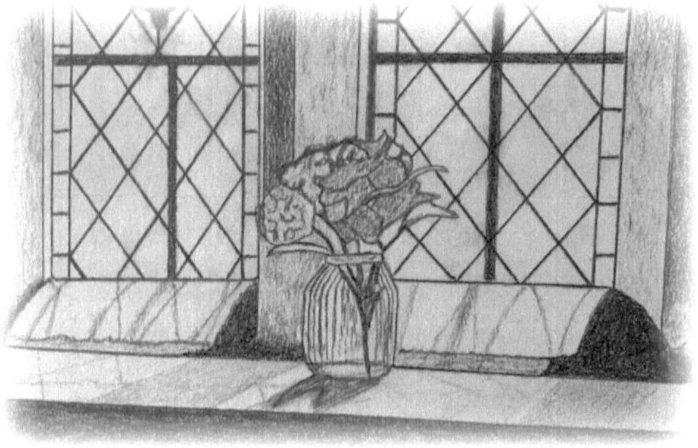

Educate. Empathy. Establish.

Recently I was asked to share "my secret" to surviving an unexpected life challenge. I hadn't really thought I was doing anything extraordinary or different than in the past. However, this person felt I had changed. I was moving through life differently. More serenely. Well, that conversation set off another journey of self-discovery for me. Was I really moving through life's uncertainty and hardships differently or was I a serenity fraud? I knew how I had tackled life's challenges in the past and the pain that ensued because of that approach, but recently I had felt more of an evolution happening within me too. Maybe I wasn't faking it after all. I began to wonder if all of the previous self-improvement work I had been doing was actually creating within me a new way of doing things. Let me share what I uncovered.

Educate. To start with, I love learning. By nature, I am a curious person who treasures the opportunity to increase my knowledge and awareness. Whether I am in a college classroom, the school of hard knocks or meditating in the classroom of silence, I find great joy in whatever desk I am sitting in. For example, I recently battled renal cancer. I won't lie, going through a significant health event was a big deal for me. It was unexpected, emergent and quite painful at times. But intertwined with those trials were also many treasures. I was surrounded by the most loving family members and healthcare staff. It may sound strange, but I was truly blessed. I did, however, feel a very strong internal pull to learn as much as I could about renal cancer, from the experts. I must repeat, to educate myself from experts. My oncologist cautioned me to not begin random internet searches that had the potential to take me down too many dark, fear-based portals. Instead, he encouraged me to seek out information from validated experts, credited by reliable sources. Such great advice!

You see, I read somewhere, the more you know, the less you will fear. I actually believe that is true, my friends, at least in my life. Think about it. The more you understand your personal situation, the less likely you are to live in fear. Apply it to your career as well. The more you understand about patient care, treatment options or anesthetic choices you may be less likely to fear that particular situation when it arises. Education helps you feel prepared, confident. It's not the only piece of my formula though. Onward, my friends.

Empathy. It took a little more soul searching, but I eventually uncovered the second piece of my life's formula, empathy. Empathy, as in a deeper connection to others through one's feelings and thoughts. Question is, how do we get there? Well, I believe part of that journey is through education and life experiences. Yes, I truly believe allowing those components to play out in your life can lead you to a more empathic living space. It may not be the only way to attain true empathy but those elements can certainly help you get started. Leaning into empathy during my cancer recovery certainly softened the experience for me. Being more empathetic towards myself and others always seems to bring out serenity in my life too. Again, not the only way to arrive, but definitely one of the tools I use to get there.

Just think about applying more empathy to your healthcare profession. What if you have a patient who presents with extreme anxiety? What about someone diagnosed with Autism Spectrum Disorder, ASD? What about a patient who is challenged with Diabetes or Parkinson's? It would make sense that we educate ourselves on those topics all the while leading with an open heart. A heart open to understanding. A heart open to empathy. If you find that empathy's arrival time is delayed, just be patient but please don't quit or turn around. I've discovered that sometimes empathy even arrives before education does. Other times, empathy is the last to arrive. What's important is that the healing grace of empathy does arrive.

I think it is also important to note that empathy is not the same as sympathy. I love how Brene' Brown explains the two terms. Brene' believes that empathy fuels connection, sympathy drives disconnection.[12] Think about it. When you stand empathically with someone, you are connecting to them. You are not judging them. You are sharing a very vulnerable moment with that person. When I am coming from a space of sympathy, for me, it's much more superficial. I'm there, but I'm not really connecting with the other person. Sometimes it's because I truly don't know what they are going through. I just can't relate. Other times, it may be because I need to protect myself from the depth of someone else's pain. Sadly, sometimes it's because I'm just too selfish to really open myself up to someone else's circumstances. Either way, I long to choose empathy. That is my intention. I invite you to make that choice with me as well.

[12] https://twentyonetoys.com/blogs/teaching-empathy/brene-brown-empathy-vs-sympathy

Establish. On to the third piece of my life's puzzle. Establishing as in "boundaries." I love this topic although it has taken me years to really unwrap it. For me, boundaries are healthy and mobile actions I take to help create a more serene life. For me, living a more educated and empathic life helped lead me into learning how to establish healthy boundaries. Boundaries like prioritizing meditation, rest and exercise in my life. Boundaries that help me to discern when I can help or when I need to volunteer at another time. The unfolding of boundary setting just didn't happen overnight though. Stay with me.

When I first began to realize the need for boundaries in my life, I went all in. Unfortunately, I got the creation of a boundary confused with the construction of a wall. At the time, my life's pendulum went from the extreme of being wishy-washy all the way to setting up unmovable concreate barriers. What I began to notice is that when I put up concrete walls, they always felt very permanent. And they were. Those walls were very hard to take down or even move. Please note though. I strongly believe there are circumstances in life that it is necessary to maintain a permanent wall of safety. If you have a co-worker who displays bullying behavior. You may need to create a wall of emotional safety. If you have a home situation where you are not physically safe, you may need to reach out for help and create a wall of safety around you. Walls are absolutely necessary, it's just they are not always needed.

So when is the creation of a boundary in your life more appropriate? When would a more adjustable action be required to help you maintain a more serene life? Let me give you some examples. Your coworkers love to go out to the bar once a week. You just happen to not like that scene. Putting up a wall would be to communicate that you would never go out with them. Putting up a boundary would be to share that the bar scene is not usually your thing. If they would be interested in doing a movie night, you would love that.

Another example might look like this: You have a very difficult patient. Someone who lives with a negative outlook, high anxiety and a general challenging disposition. Creating a wall would be to dismiss this patient from your practice. What if you creatively looked at this challenge instead? Decided to schedule this particular patient first thing in the morning so you wouldn't have to dread the rest of the day. That could actually be a blessing for the patient as well, especially if anxiety is a challenge for them. Maybe your staff takes turns working with this person. Share the challenges. Notice, I'm not encouraging you to hold gossip sessions where hurtful opinions are shared and judgment is passed. Rather, respectfully communicate these challenges with a trusted coworker who is willing to creatively brainstorm solutions. I believe that working and living this way does not make you indecisive, rather it empowers you to live more confidently, less fearfully, more fluidly. Boundaries are beautiful.

So, try this out. If something is bothering you, educate yourself first. See if that leads to a more empathetic space of understanding which could ultimately allow you to establish healthy boundaries if needed. Educate. Empathy. Establish. Triple E. Could it really be that easy? Why not give it a try and then decide.

Reflection:

Is there an area of your life that you are struggling with? Is there a work issue or a personal challenge that is eliciting fear and frustration inside you? Consider educating yourself on this topic. You can begin by searching out reliable sources. Check your community library for the material. Contact a supportive agency that may offer you material. Begin educating yourself on this topic and see if empathy and established boundaries begin to flow from your heart. You are worth it!

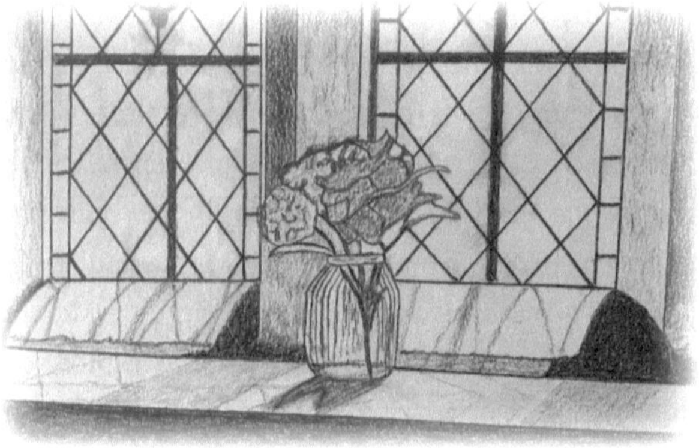

Reaching Out

When I keep my heart in the lead, I reach out more than I reach in, my soul is at peace. When I see others reaching outward, instead of inwardly focused, that inspires me too. I'm not talking about living life as a martyr to the point of exhaustion or manipulating others around you in order to look good. I'm talking about true, genuine selfish-less acts of kindness. Humans with their hearts and arms stretched wide open. Could there be anything more inspiring, more beautiful to witness? Not in my world. Well, except maybe the face of a grandchild, but that's another book.

So what does reaching out look like for you, for me? Can it really impact your life in a positive way? Honestly, answering those questions can get a little tricky. I'm wondering if many of us in healthcare are already "reaching out superstars." Reaching out might even be one of our superpowers. Maybe reaching out is already built right into our chosen careers. Maybe it's not. If it is, reading this may even seem unnecessary. Either way, I urge you to stay with me. There is always the chance you could explore different avenues to help you grow your reaching-outward muscle. From surprising someone with a bouquet of flowers to helping rebuild someone's home after a flood. When an act of kindness originates in the heart, it has the power to change a life, to change our world. And our world sure needs it.

So where to begin exploring the aspect of reaching out. How do we discover that if we're already tapped out or have very little time, energy or heart to reach out? Could we plug in our Triple E theory? Educate, empathize and establish boundaries? Why not. For me, it was actually that process that helped me discern my path forward. It helped me navigate my successes and failures along my reaching out journey. And I must share, even my failures, were pure joy when reaching out to others and sharing my heart/talents with them. If your heart is open, may I offer a few learnings I stumbled upon with the hope of sparking an avenue of outreach in your life? My intention, though, is to help you get your creative wheels turning not to toot my own horn.

What I humbly recommend you do is begin with things you already enjoy. No this is not an act of selfishness, it's just a springboard for you to begin somewhere. Are you more comfortable around adults or children? If you enjoy adults, try connecting to a senior assisted living facility in your community. Years ago, after listening to a wonderful speaker at a continuing education program, I felt compelled to contact my community's senior living complex. I connected with a nurse who worked there. She informed me that every resident they served was expected to receive oral care, every day, by a staff member. What I began to wonder was how much oral care training did those staff members receive. I decided to try and create a training program that could become an oral care resource for every employee. I must admit, it was tricky working around the different shifts each employee worked but I persisted. As it turned out, teaching the lead nurse and a few employees how to provide thorough and gentle oral care to their residents was enough to begin this effort. I hope, in the long term, it helped serve both workers and residents.

If you do enjoy serving the adult population, what about volunteering to become a Senior Services volunteer transportation driver? My oldest daughter chose to provide this simple act of service for several years. Just once a week, for a few hours, she helps transport seniors around our small community. Another daughter volunteered at a Hospice home, another daughter mentors an adolescent, while another daughter reaches out to elementary children during their lunch hour. I've even been blessed to watch my husband volunteer with Youth Outreach teams that serve others by doing home improvement projects of all different skill levels. I'm not sure who is more blessed, the recipients or the giver, but I love seeing the fruits of those interactions changing our world for the better.

For me, the acts of service I enjoy the most involve the preschool population. I believe many dental practitioners can relate to the deep sadness we feel when listening to a child cry while receiving restorative work. It doesn't happen much anymore due to the safe use of Nitrous Oxide and other dental strategies, but I can still remember those cries. Rather than allowing that memory to fester, I allowed it to propel me to reach out to area preschools. I stopped asking "why" was that happening" and started asking "what" could I do about it. Talk about empowering! For 10 years and counting, I have shared a simple, fun, interactive dental program with preschool children in my community. This time has been a treasured memory for me. It is also with great hope that I have planted the seeds of dental health in our younger population…one smile at a time.

There is another group of beautiful humans that I have also enjoyed serving. For almost 14 years, I have volunteered monthly with a group of adults with differing abilities. This gathering happens under the umbrella of my faith organization but it has traveled out into the community as well. The program has grown in ways I never would have imagined. Interesting how my two favorite acts of service have spilled over into my professional life. I volunteer on my own time, both the preschool and the differing abilities groups but the fruits of these opportunities have certainly overlapped into my professional life. I love seeing the faces of those I volunteered with walking through my operatory doors. Those are some of my best days!

So where and how do you want to share your smile? Go on a healthcare mission trip. Write a simple article for your local newspaper on the topic of health and wellbeing. Support the staff at an area nursing home. Develop dental and or health programs to bring into your school systems. Be committed to writing and posting positive dental Facebook and/or Twitter posts. Feel where your heart is leading you and then go for it. Reach out! We need you! Our world is waiting!

Reflection:

If you already volunteer, continue that generous act of service. If you are waiting to get started, connect with a local agency and commit to exploring the possibility of serving. You can make a phone call, go online or meet another volunteer for coffee to begin this journey. Emphasis on the word "begin." It doesn't matter how fast you get there. Forward is forward. And you remember, you are worth it!

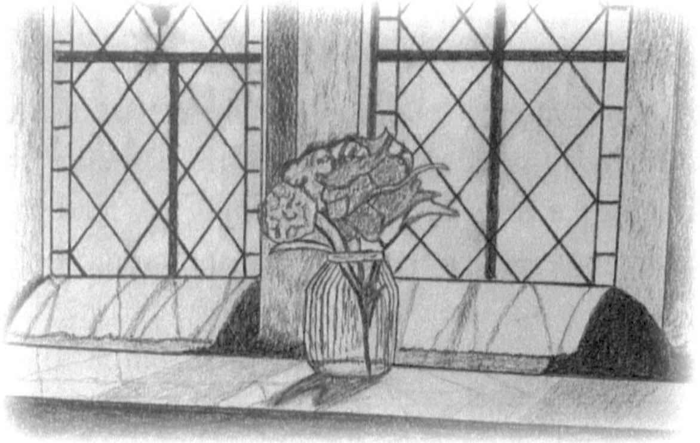

I Am Not Afraid of Storms, for I Am Learning How to Sail My Ship

Louisa May Alcott

I believe that everyone reading this book can relate to moments, even seasons, of hardship and grief. Although we hold different deposits in our memory banks of these events, nevertheless, the memories are a part of us. For me, sometimes the hardest memories have changed me the most. I don't fear them anymore. I don't repress them anymore. I honor them.

Working in the healthcare profession, while dealing with personal grief and hardships, is not an easy road for anyone to travel down. Personally, I've had to seek supportive measures when dealing with these issues. Measures that included professional counseling services, short term time absence from my job, lightening my load at home, reaching out to friends more often and even simply making sure I was getting sleep, exercise and eating balanced meals. Did I do all this perfectly? Far from it. There were times I showed up to work, smiling on the outside but a train wreck on the inside. Can you relate? If so, you can identify with the enormous strength it requires to work while dealing with hardship and grief. But it can be done. Don't isolate yourself though. Reach out and get some help. Let your employer and/or office manager know what is happening in your life. Have courage. Have compassion and know you are not alone.

I also long to honor the challenges our healthcare patients are dealing with. Some carry heavy burdens that are more visible and others, invisible baggage. Whether you can see their grief, I believe we need a tender touch when working with all our patients. Those who have lost loved ones, suffered job losses, dealing with any number of mental health issues or carrying baggage from their past that weighs them down. Please don't back away from their discomfort. You don't have to join someone on their journey but you can absolutely recognize it, honor it and offer your support and understanding. Sometimes just leaning in, making eye contact and listening attentively can communicate genuine care and concern to another soul. Again, leaning in with empathy and not just sympathy.

What I'd also like to share next might seem trivial to you but trust me, it is far from inconsequential. The memory did surprise me though. I was hoping for some profound, life-changing moment to share with you to elaborate on my thoughts. But true to my learning style, it was a diamond in the rough of memories from my sister's struggle with cancer that embellished this memory. Today I can still vividly remember the tears flowing from my eyes as I listened to my sister share how isolated she felt on her cancer journey. One would have never guessed that. She was surrounded, almost guarded, by a very loving family. A love that never wavered. Yet she longed for friendships that could go the distance with her. Friendships not afraid to journey down the hard road of cancer and its ensuing hardships. She even ached for "routine" medical and/or dental appointments. I know everyone did their best to meet her needs, but in reality, it wasn't enough. She needed more "normal." And that, my friend, is sometimes where we, the healthcare profession can fill in a gap.

So how do we bring normal into our healthcare practices when dealing with patients who have been stripped of their normal? Recognizing this challenge prompted me to evaluate how I really serve and treat my patients. Do I separate myself from them or do I have the courage it takes to join them, to connect with them? There are some patients who come to us suffering great hardships. Others are dealing with short-term discomfort. Patients and their families who don't want to be coddled or treated like children, but do need a higher level of compassionate care. Patients who long to be treated like they were before their challenging journey began. Patients who are fighting to hold onto their "normal."

This is the authentic space I want you to challenge yourself to enter into. A space that just doesn't feel sacred, it is sacred. In that sweet veil of grace remember to treat all your patients with kindness and respect but please allow for a little extra compassion when working with anyone struggling with grief. That patient might present with less than standard home care efforts. Your patient may be quieter or even the opposite, more talkative. Either way, refrain from scolding someone who is suffering. That, my friend, only adds salt to a very painful wound. If you can, try and connect with them at some level. Reassuring them they are not alone.

I also find it very respectful to show your full attention with everyone your serve. Whether it is a coworker, family, friend or patient. Try to slow down enough to maintain eye contact. This is a hard one for me. I can multi-task with the best but that is not what is most needed when working with someone who is suffering. When a patient is sharing with you their challenging medical update or life story please don't move around the room. Sit still. Take notes. Devote yourself to the human you are with.

If you're like me, you may also need to really dig deep into your listening skills. Try to reflect part of someone's story back to them. Even if you can't relate to their experience, but simply reflecting what you've heard is a very tender courtesy. This kindness shows someone they were heard. And in my world, being heard can also communicate that I've been seen. I no longer exist on a deserted island of isolation and pain.

I wonder if you could also offer extra comfort adjuncts but respect your patient if they decline those options. A simple neck pillow or blanket can help a patient feel comforted and not compromised. Bringing in a more comfortable chair is also another option. Just try and follow your patient's lead. If they are upbeat and stoic, I encourage you to mirror that. If there are tears escaping their eyes, allow the space for that to happen. Try to be fully present no matter what you do. It is a priceless gift with no expiration date.

And finally, please make sure you keep your patient, friend or family member on your calendar, if they wish to be, regardless of their prognosis. We all long for hope. Please don't be the person to take that priceless gift of hope away from anyone. And when the time comes, when they leave this earth, I encourage you to find a way to attend a funeral service or commemoration service. Yes, out of respect for the beautiful life you were a part of, but also for yourself. If you give yourself wholeheartedly to your profession, you are going to experience loss. I hope, by whatever action you take, you can find a way to process your feelings. You will bring honor to your patient when you do so. What a beautiful expression of respect and love you will be offering to the universe.

Reflection:

Find some quiet time to reflect on your mental health at this present moment. If you are balanced, lean into that balance. If you are dealing with hardship or grief, journal what is happening and how you are feeling. If need be, consider reaching out to a friend, co-worker or counselor to help wrap love and support around you. Trust me. You won't regret this action. Anytime you invite others to your "island," healing is there waiting for you. And remember, you are worth it.

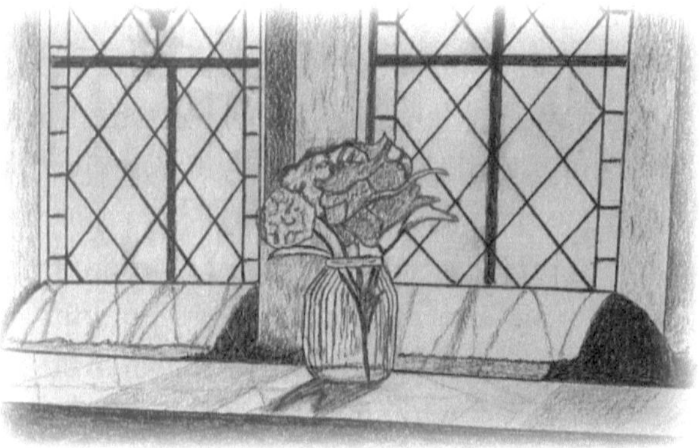

Staying Sustainable

Whenever I hear the word sustainable, I break out and smile. Probably not hard for you to imagine a dental hygienist breaking out in a smile but I'm serious. Even my listening skills go on high alert and my focus becomes even more tuned in. You see, deep down, even before that phrase became popular, I believe sustainability was in my soul. It wasn't just my face that would smile, my soul always lit up too. Before I could even identify sustainable actions, I seemed to always gravitate towards reducing, reusing and recycling. Some of those actions were based on necessity. When I was a child, as well as raising my own children, we lived a very sustainable life. We tried hard not to waste anything. To share with others what we had and somehow, there was always enough.

You know, looking back, I'm so thankful I was raised to respect the world around me by living more sustainably. Were we perfect? Was I perfect? Absolutely not. But I believe in progress, not perfection. I believe in moving forward. I believe in the family, the community and the planet I am a part of. Sustainability. Going Green. Reduce. Reuse. Recycle. Environmentally friendly. Reduce your carbon footprint. Sharing the love. They are all wonderful catchphrases that can point us to a universal concept in our personal life, just stay with me. It's going to be fun.

Most recently I've spent a lot of time reflecting on some of the sustainable actions that spilled out around me during the Covid 19 Pandemic. From grocery shopping online to Zoom birthday parties to learning how to not waste a pinch of anything in your pantry. Sustainability was sure happening in my world. It may have played out differently in your space but I truly believe the underlying current of sustainability was there for all of us. We had to quickly learn another way of living. And hopefully, a healthier way of moving in our world at home and at work.

One thing I began to notice during the Covid 19 pandemic was the crowds of humans working from home. I wonder how many other healthcare workers noticed the effect this had on vehicle traffic to and from work. I won't lie, I loved it. Although it was a significant challenge for many who had to creatively transition to work from home, everyone agreed this simple action began to significantly reduce car emissions and other environmental effects vehicles had on our planet. I imagine if the earth could talk, or in this case shout, we would have all heard a breathless, "thank you!"

I wonder if anyone else noticed how many more people were spending more time outdoors, walking, biking, or hiking. Maybe you found yourself rediscovering a community nature trail as I did. Maybe you pumped up your bike tires and began peddling around your neighborhood more. Maybe all you could do was get yourself to and from work without physically, emotionally or mentally collapsing. So many brave healthcare workers stood guard and protected us all and we will be forever grateful for your sacrifice. From my heart to yours, thank you!

Yes, there were challenges but there were also many blessings. It was so humbling to witness the wonderful outpouring of acts of kindness spilling out around us. We all learned to get creative and stretchy in order to find solutions. And you know what? I believe we did it! I'm not saying that everything we had to modify during the Covid pandemic had healthy outcomes but I do believe we all showed up and gave it our best effort. And you know me, I'm always looking for the silver, sustainable linings.

I also realize there was tremendous turmoil going on all around us during this pandemic. Hopefully, when this book goes to print, those significant challenges will be behind us. Either way, there is so much for us to learn from. I know I have certainly adapted how I move in this world. I'm hopeful these changes have had a positive effect on our planet and ultimately those living on it as well. Even when the Covid 19 pandemic is in our rear-view mirror, I believe we'll need to continually evaluate our carbon footprint with every step. And why not? These simple actions don't even need to be complicated. We do need to do our part though.

For me, I believe the concept of sustainability can positively and simply impact the way we live, work and play regardless if we're living during a pandemic. This term is much more than just being "green" or environmentally friendly." It entails looking at the entire picture. People, planet and profit. To be sustainable is to "meet the needs of the present without compromising the ability of future generations to meet their own needs." (World Commission on Environment and Development.)[13] I still get very excited whenever I think of reducing my carbon footprint or accessing my environmental impact. Every time I look into the eyes of a child, I feel a commitment to their future as well as my own.

I'm curious how many readers practice home recycling. I have a feeling we're all engaged at some level with this practice. What about your professional life? Do you

[13] https://stats.oecd.org/glossary/detail.asp?ID=2626

recycle at work? Five years ago, my work environment did not. I'm happy to say that we are all on board today by tapping into our community recycling program. If you're interested in starting a recycling program at your place of employment why not contact your local Recycling Center first. Check out if they have a recycling program you could join. Trust me on this. You won't regret it.

I'm thankful our office did just that. To date, we fill up three, 95-gallon recycling bins every month. Our bins are picked up monthly. Doing a little simple math, this means we save close to 3,420 gallons of waste annually. Waste that is recycled and not added to our local landfill. We are also cognizant of product duplication. We think before we order. We attempt to cluster our orders or purchase in bulk to help reduce the automobile traffic needed to deliver these products.

What about your office lighting? Can you contact a local electrician to have them evaluate your light sources? How environmentally effective is your lighting? How cost-effective would it be to improve those elements? Why not solicit help from your coworkers? We are always stronger together. I personally found it very humbling to see others re-evaluating their practices and implementing more sustainable actions in their work space too. They thought of things I never would have. Did it impact me and my workflow? Yes, it did, but it was so worth the minor changes I needed to incur to reduce our carbon footprints.

I think we also need to pause here to mention the critical need to guard all personal and patient protection practices we already have in play. By no means am I asking you to jeopardize anyone's safety. I am personally blessed to work in an environment where personal and patient safety is paramount. When it comes to sterilization procedures and other protective barriers, you can't cut corners. But you can collectively brainstorm other ways to reduce your environmental impact without reducing safety. Trust me, it can be done and done now, not later. Get a team together at work to either begin a sustainability program or join a team already in place. You will never regret being a part of this effort.

A few more quick thoughts. Do you live close enough to bike to work or even walk to work? Talk about arriving fresh and ready to go after your morning commute. What about carpooling? Do you live nearby another co-worker that you could share a ride with? These are just a sprinkling of ideas to get you thinking about helping you and your healthcare practice become more sustainable. I haven't seen this yet, but I also dream of seeing individual wind turbines connected to healthcare offices. I would love to see roof solar panels in place as well. Not only would we be reducing our carbon footprint but think of the reduction of dependence you would have with your power supply company. A trifecta in the world of sustainability.

Do I think this will all happen overnight? Of course not. I personally still muddle through most of my days but my heart is always focused on moving sustainably in my world. I hope you too can look into the eyes of a child and commit to them your best. Commit to living and working in a way that will help create and sustain a beautiful world for them to grow old in. We're in this together friend. Let the wind turbines of knowledge continue to circulate in our world and in our lives. Let those winds blow healing and continued health in our world.

Reflection:

What is one simple action (or reduction of an action) that you can take to positively impact our planet? It can be as simple as searching online for ways to begin this journey. How about choosing fabric napkins instead of paper napkins? Volunteer at your local recycling center. How about learning more about Wind Turbines? What about contacting a government representative to view their stance on environmental impact. Are you the team member to bring a recycling program to your place of employment? Whatever you do, I urge you to take one small action today and see where that leads you. Remember, you and the next generations are so worth it!

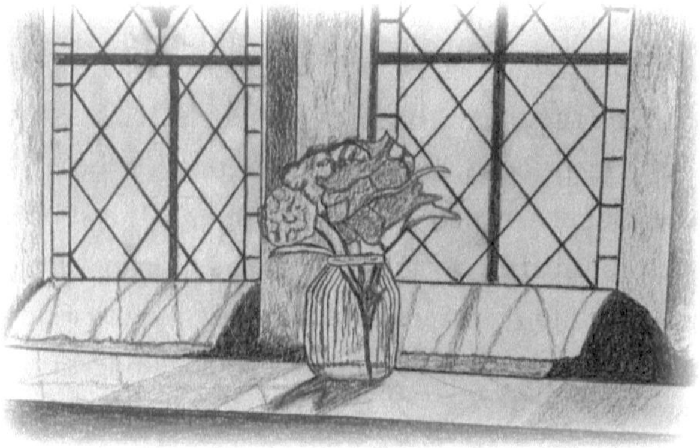

Foundation Built on a Shop Floor

I've experienced the joy of a very interesting employment history. Believe it or not, I've gone from working in the machine tool and die industry to the dental hygiene profession. Quite the jump isn't it? I've gone from smelling grease and machine exhaust to smelling antiseptics, dental cements and an assortment of other dental products. Even within the career of dental hygiene, I've experienced a wonderful degree of variation too. But let's not skip too far ahead yet. As with every person on this planet, every structure built, every nation, every mountain, I believe it all exists because of its foundation. For me, before I could lean into the many blessings of my healthcare career, I needed to pay homage to the foundation that has helped sustain me these past 40 years.

As I mentioned, my careeer foundation began in my parents' family-owned machine tool and die shop which they established in 1976, and of which I am very proud. With five children under their roof, my father's many years of experience, his tenacity and my mother's devotion, they opened the doors to a family-run business that continues to operate today. At first, I was thrilled with this family adventure. I even have a copy of the "For Sale" sign that came off the building. I was so geeked about the experience that I made a copy of that sign using the company's first copy machine. Don't laugh, but it's still tucked away in a childhood scrapbook somewhere in my basement.

However, when the honeymoon wore off and I began sweeping metal curls off the shop floor, painting machines a lovely shade of gray and eventually learning how to run a small drill press I was a tad embarrassed and exhausted. I was a teenager not wanting to sport grease under my fingernails, strap on metal-toed boots or wear fashionable eye safety glasses. Let's also be honest. I might have carried a wee bit of teenage attitude with me as well. Either way, I was so very proud of my parents and thankful for the chance to earn some spending money. It was a very interesting time in my life. Little did I know, these strong work ethics would become a part of my durable foundation in the years to come. I am so very grateful for every opportunity my parents provided me, even the greasy fingernails.

And there have definitely been many more years spent in the workforce that I have been immensely thankful for the work values that were instilled in me while working in a machine shop. I was 19 when I graduated from dental hygiene school and began to work in the dental field. I've spent the majority of those years in private practice but I've also had the blessing of working in a Native American Tribal Dental Clinic, the hygiene clinic at a local Community College, became a feature writer for *RDH* magazine and had the blessing of volunteering/serving the community in which I live in. I have loved and learned from it all.

My time working in a Native American Dental Clinic was incredible. I worked with a wonderful dentist who encouraged me to expand my skills and knowledge. He helped me establish a school-based community fluoridation program. He also encouraged me to begin digging into, forgive the pun, the world of periodontics. I was also welcomed into the beautiful Native American culture. A culture I have such great respect for. To this day, I must admit that I also had one of the most beautiful views out my operatory window while I worked at that dental clinic. Not to make you jealous, but I gazed out onto an expansive fresh water bay that made the stress of a person's dental schedule just melt off your shoulders. If I close my eyes, I can still see the glitter of the sun dancing on that expanse of water. When I meditate, that is often one of my "happy places" my imagination takes me to. Trust me, you'd want to go too.

My learning opportunities working in the Dental Hygiene Clinic at a local community college were also incredible. I must admit that one of my greatest take-aways from that experience was learning to deal with my fears, especially the fear of not being good enough. Just the courage it took for me to leave my comfortable wheel-house of private practice was huge. What I discovered was priceless! This learning institution housed a plethora of clinicians eager to help me become my best. Clinicians that were not looking for me to be perfect. Clinicians that allowed me to grow professionally and also for me to help others do the same. I will be forever thankful for the years I spent in that portal of learning.

I am also eternally grateful for the many opportunities I've experienced in private practice. But what takes up the most space in my heart are the co-workers and dental patients I served during that time. The relationships I have built will sustain me forever. I personally think it's one of many unsung perks of private practice. You have the honor of generally seeing your patients at least twice a year for as long as they are connected to your dental practice. That, my friend, can be very special. To me, the best example I have of this blessing is when the next generation dental patient comes in to see you. That is so humbling and rewarding all at the same time.

In my opinion, I don't think any of these opportunities can happen if your ego gets in the way. Whatever healthcare setting you are working in. Whether you are working with a dental patient or a co-worker, if your ego shows up first, gets defensive, the likelihood of befuddling the relationship dramatically increases. Do yourself a favor. When you get to work, purpose to leave your ego in the car. You won't regret it. If you really want to elevate your healthcare career to more than an eight to five job, you must surrender your ego in order to receive the many blessings waiting for you. Whatever environment you work in, leave your ego home!

I'd also like to share with you a career tangent that arrived in my life a few years back. Sprinkled in my private practice career was the discovery of the *RDH* magazine. Actually, it was more like a re-introduction. I had been a closet fan of *RDH* magazine for years. There have been, and continue to be many writers that are responsible for filling up my bucket when it dries up. Again, I took another huge leap of faith connecting to the Editor of *RDH* with my first submission. I'm so thankful I did. I discovered another wonderful group of colleagues that also wanted the best for me while allowing me to filter my thoughts back out into the dental community. So many blessings continue to flow from all of my work experiences.

What about you? What does your career foundation look like? Has it been built well or do you need to shore things up a bit? Are you someone who is dependable, reliable, a team player? Or do you struggle with some of those issues? You know, it is never too late to begin building stronger work ethics, to work on your foundation. Maybe you would be more successful with a different work environment? Maybe it's your home environment that is affecting your work commitments. Maybe there are some personal issues you need to deal with. Don't be afraid to expose those challenges, bring them out in the open. Once you can logically look at a situation, many times a solution will present itself. The trick is, you need to bring it out into the open.

I can't promise you a bed of roses while you're at work, or a shop floor covered in metal curlings either. What I can do, is hope that you will encounter more job satisfaction that pours from consistent and reliable work ethics and behaviors. Build your foundation on the solid ground, my friend. You won't regret it, especially when encountering obstacles such as a global pandemic. You'll be able to lean into the unknown and stand firm on your work foundation, even if you temporarily have to stand on the sidelines. Nothing in life is ever wasted, my friend. Nothing!

Reflection:

Pack yourself some courage and honestly evaluate your work ethics and values. Are you reliable? Are you able to give your best while you are at work? Are there some obstacles that prevent you from doing that? Are there any amends you need to make to past employers or coworkers? Don't go at this list alone. Find a trusted friend, share your findings and then make a plan to move forward. I promise you won't regret it because you are so worth it!

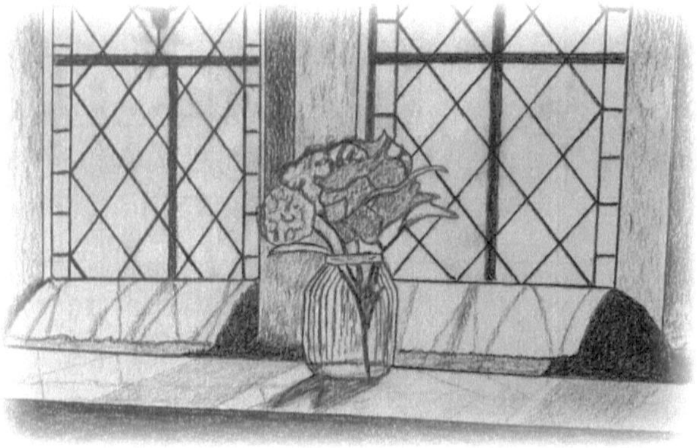

Pay For Health or Health Care

This can be a very touchy subject. Paying for health or waiting to pay for health care. I learned that lesson early on when a co-worker responded to my grumbling over the cost of a gym membership. I was just commenting that I longed to establish a more regular exercise routine but didn't have the finances to pay for some of the more elite memberships. Thankfully she didn't argue with me or pile shame into my soul. She just very simply stated that sometimes in life you have to pay for health or you will later pay for health care. Make the choice.

This response stopped me in my tracks. She was right. Paying for that gym membership vs waiting for my health to lessen was true wisdom. I believe that philosophy has absolutely aided my overall health, maybe even helped push off a diagnosis of diabetes that is riddled in my family history. I also believe my decade's commitment to yoga practice has also helped sustain my healthcare career for almost 40 years. However, some of these preventative health modalities have a financial cost to them, some have a time management restraint, yet some can now be found absolutely free. Personally, I think it all comes down to loving yourself enough and choosing to prioritize healthy choices. I'm not saying it will be easy, I'm just saying it will be worth it.

I must confess that I am preaching to my own choir of challenges though. I didn't always prioritize regular exercise. There were many years I considered that running after my four children was exercise enough. Looking back, I realize I was doing the best I could at the time but I was always feeling drawn to a healthier lifestyle. It just took me a while, but once I found my niche, there was no stopping me. I found some very creative ways to incorporate healthy living all the while balancing my finances and time challenges. And I loved it! When I didn't have the extra finances I learned that walking the circumference of a shopping mall could be very effective and easy to do. It was even more fun when others joined me, or maybe it was me joining them? Not sure which came first but I loved that season in my life.

In some ways, exercise became like a hobby for me. I began to really enjoy all aspects of physical movement. From outdoor bike riding, mall walking and eventually joining a gym. It was all good. My love affair with physical exercise really suffered a blow though when my exercise classes and routines were temporarily closed during the Covid 19 pandemic. Oh my heart, did I ever miss it! Although I did create an at-home workout routine and schedule, it just wasn't the same for me. On the flip side of this challenge, I did hear some people found home workouts that really benefited them during this time in history. Guess it just validates that, with exercise, there is definitely not a one-size-fits-all. What matters most is that you keep trying, keep showing up.

I need to get really honest with you right now though. I wish I could say that this philosophy eliminated the need for health care in my life. It didn't. Life can still get messy, turn on a dime. I do, however, believe my commitment to a healthy lifestyle strengthened me for the journey I am now on. I have recently been diagnosed with Stage 2 Renal Cell Carcinoma. After the emergent removal of my right kidney and cancerous tumor, I began my journey of recovery. I truly believe because I was so committed to an exercise routine, yoga practice, meditation and a strong spiritual practice my recovery is headed in the right direction. I was able to return to my beloved career and family life with a hopeful and positive future, cancer-free. I am a walking miracle!

I truly hope and pray that sharing my story will spark, or continue lighting, a healthy workout routine in your life. I am now living proof that there are no guarantees in life. Even if we are preventively focused, the storm clouds of illness can settle over us. But who knows, maybe our recovery from such illnesses will be shortened because of our pre-commitment to exercise and other healthy choices. On a very positive note, maybe our healthy lifestyle will positively influence others along our journey too. I truly believe, if you look deep enough, you'll find a silver lining in any cloud. And who knows, maybe even a rainbow or two.

Reflection:

Is there an area of your life that challenges your overall health? Food choices? Exercise program? Sleep habits? Meditation practice or lack of one. Just identify one aspect and break it down into steps. If there is a financial barrier, see if you can adjust your budget in other areas in order to afford the cost. If there is a time barrier, break that down too. You might be surprised to discover how little increments of time add up over time. And always remember, you are worth it!

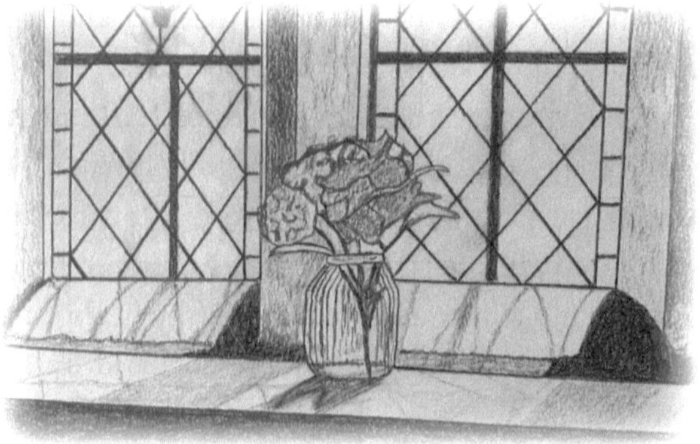

Want to Find the Magic?

I've heard it said that stepping out of your comfort zone is where magic can happen. The trick is finding the courage to make that leap.

I believe every human, in one way or another, longs to find their personal magic zone. I believe we all have those dreams. Some dreams just have a few more road-blocks to navigate before reaching that place of fulfillment. That's just life. There could be financial challenges, learning challenges, medical hardships or any number of life constraints. Whatever barrier you may be facing that is preventing you from making that leap I want you to first have the courage to identify it and then make a choice to deal with it. So let's first get brave together and begin to identify and unpack some of those obstacles.

For me, I've seen the challenges of fear and anxiety negatively play out in my life especially after my sister's passing at age 45. I found myself trying to care for my own four children plus help with her three children. Trying to balance home, family and working in the healthcare field began to take a toll on me. I was so focused on helping others through grief that I had not allowed myself to journey through it. It was only a few months after her passing that life started to catch up with me. Although I projected an "everything is ok" attitude on the outside, inside I was a mess. I wasn't sleeping well. I was overwhelmed just thinking about the next day and I also began to show physical symptoms of my grief. Truthfully, I felt completely void of any magic, anywhere in my soul.

When my body's battle cry finally caught my attention, I sought out a wonderful grief support group that began to help me heal. This circle of like-minded souls allowed me to open up, in a safe space, with no judgment. Especially without a little one's eyes watching me cry my heart out. A space of rest. A space of comfort where I could reorientate myself and begin to heal.

Along this journey of discovery, little sparks of light began finding their way into my soul. I began volunteering at a Hospice Home. For me, the magic of healing really started unfolding in that space. It was a gradual heal, as most wounds are, but healing was happening especially when I could offer my love and support to another grieving family. What is it about the magic of receiving a gift only to give it away? I don't know how it works, I can only testify that it worked for me.

If you've been able to unpack some of your barriers, are you ready for some magic? Let's circle back to stepping out of our comfort zones and into spaces where beauty and authenticity happen. That is the space I finally found myself in that helped re-open my desire to write. Truth was, part of me always wanted to be a writer. Nothing full-time. Just an avenue to capture my love for the healthcare profession and other thoughts I have. I had even visualized myself as I writer for years. I had just gotten a little lost along the way. Lost in my fears of taking risks. Lost in exhaustion. What about you? Has anything popped up in your heart? Any sparks of magic beginning to surface?

Well, for me as I worked through this process of healing, I began gleaning a bit of courage and stopped coming up with excuses why I couldn't write and just started writing. I had the courage to finally explore writing for the *RDH* magazine. I was finally beginning to uncover the roadblocks that were keeping me from reaching my potential. Roadblocks that were keeping me stuck in my comfort zone, away from the magic. I'm wondering if that is beginning to happen in your life.

You see, for me, it can be just as heartbreaking to see others experience those challenges too. I'm thinking of you. Someone I'll probably never meet yet someone I already hope will be guided gently into their space of living more fully. Someone brave enough to identify barriers and willing to dangle their toes outside of their comfort zone. Someone ready to become their more genuine self.

If you still find yourself stuck in a personal barrier though, I want you to know you aren't alone. Today we have wonderful support adjuncts available to address any challenge. There are personal counselors, self-help books and/or support groups. Is it scary to seek help? It might be. Is it worth it? I believe it is priceless! Do you have to do it alone? Absolutely not. As I just shared, I needed to lean on family members, support groups and friendships for extra encouragement to step out of my comfort zone to face the obstacles preventing me from reaching my potential. So thankful they were there for me. It would be an honor to be there for you.

So what do you think? Are you willing to open yourself up to a little magic? If you are stuck in the slow zone, if you are riddled in the fear zone just remember you aren't alone and yes, you can break through! Everything previously mentioned can absolutely help you move towards that zone where you are your most authentic self. Personally, my growth came very slowly. In fact, there were days when I felt forward momentum only to slide backward a while later. Funny thing is, as long as I continued to plug along, I was eventually catapulted forward again. Forward is forward, no matter the speed. Who knows? Your growth could happen more quickly and that's wonderful. Whatever the pace is, just be willing to want to move towards that magic zone. Just think of the possibilities. Give yourself permission to dream, to journal, to imagine what it would look and feel like to step out of your safe comfort zone. The world needs you to step out. We need magic more than we ever have. We need you! So get comfortable with being uncomfortable, because that's where the magic happens.

Reflection:

When you close your eyes and imagine yourself living your best life, what does that look like? Maybe you want to journal those ideas. Maybe you are more comfortable plotting a strategy. Developing action plans. Have you ever done any mandala work? I love using a circle to draw my feelings and dreams inside it. It's never fancy work for me. It's amazing what has come out of me though. You can encapsulate your life's dreams within that circle. You can post it or your goals and action items where you can see them every day. Allow yourself the chance to dream your way out of your comfort zone and into the magic of living your best life. You just might find those dreams will become reality too. And remember, you are worth it!

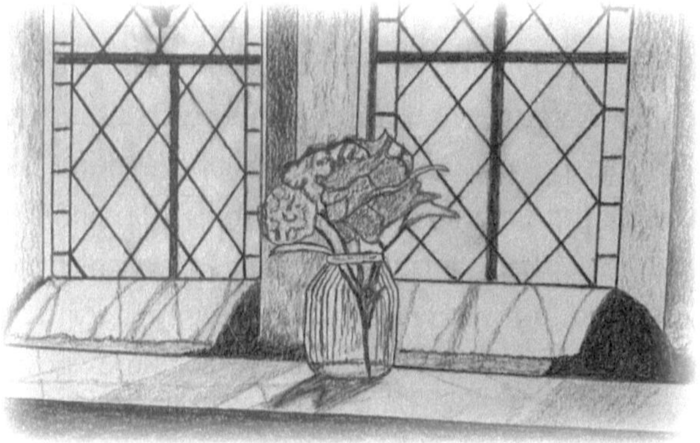

POWER OF NETWORKING

Networking is not a new cultural phenomenon. In one form or another, I'm guessing networking has been around since the beginning of human existence. It may have looked different than it does today, but it is probably even more vital now. Back during pre-historic times, I imagine early humans had to network food sources, water sources, the location of dangerous animals and even shelter options among many other survival strategies. It's been shown, on so many levels, that one of the most dangerous human behaviors is self-isolating. Simply put, we need networking in our lives in order to survive. In order to thrive. No matter what century we are in, isolating yourself can have devastating effects. We learn and grow in relationships and networking can provide that lifelong gift. Since the beginning of time, humans have relied on networking. It's just been more recently that we've put language around that phenomenon.

Before I share another personal confession (sorry) I need you to know it was never my intention to reveal so many details from my "dental diary," but here I go again: I never really understood networking early on in my career, early on in my life. Not because I chose to ignore it, but because I wasn't aware of it. You don't know, what you don't know. At the beginning of my healthcare career, I was so focused on learning new skills in school, graduating and then beginning my career. I was not wise enough to stay connected to professional organizations that would have provided me so many networking opportunities. I, more or less, set out on my employment path with my head down, my ego in the lead and determined to be as successful as possible. Problem was, I missed so much along the way! I do not recommend this approach, my friend. Thankfully, my blinders came off and I began to see the blessings that networking could provide. And not in a selfish, "what can I get out of this relationship attitude" but rather in a "how can I share and give back" way of living.

Today, networking has a very positive effect on my career and personal life. I wholeheartedly encourage you to evaluate how and if you are on a networking path. Establishing professional and personal networking relationships, whether in person or on a secured online platform. Each has the potential to open many doors for you. Had it not been for an employer making a phone call to another colleague back in 1984, I would have struggled even more finding employment in the new community I had just moved to. My employer took the time to personally reach out to someone to validate my credentials. To network on my behalf. This action opened the door for me to sub in this new community which led to many wonderful career opportunities.

Networking can easily help you reach out to other professionals for advice and encouragement, welcome others into your professional circle and eventually become a portal for others to establish their career fulfillment. So, what could that look like in your life? It could be as easy as joining your professional healthcare organization. Or, how about connecting with an online professional group such as LinkedIn? What about Social platform sites that have professional groups available for you to connect to? I need to push the pause button for a moment though. Please use caution when visiting social networking sites. Never forget for a second, that even if you are a part of a closed professional group, you still have a very public audience. Be careful what you post and/or respond to. Ok. We can push the resume button now.

What about purposing to invite other professionals out to lunch on a regular basis? This is always a win-win in my world. Wish I would have done more of this though. Lunch hours have always been so unpredictable for me that I've hesitated to try to schedule lunch meetings with other professionals. Why didn't I look for simple solutions, such as bringing a packed lunch and meeting in a park for a networking lunch, instead of dismissing the action? I know I was doing my best at that time in my life though. Just sharing a little food for thought, my friend.

What about creating a business card for you to share with other healthcare professionals at Continuing Education events. If you've done any personal branding work, this could be easily accomplished. The possibilities are endless and can certainly be tailored to your personality. If you are more introverted, connecting online may be more comfortable for you. If you are typically more extroverted you may find creating professional lunch opportunities suits your style of networking. Whatever you choose, remember to keep your conversation professional. Networking is not a platform to professionally vent or gossip about your employer or coworkers. It should be a safe place to support each other's professional development. Offer advice when you are asked, otherwise, your role could be to just listen.

I also encourage you to network outside of your healthcare circle. We don't exist in a bubble, nor should we. That space is too vulnerable and isolating as previously mentioned. Reach out to other community members. I have personally been blessed with a mentoring relationship that has lasted over 10 years and counting. After meeting someone, while volunteering, I was blessed to establish a wonderful friendship. The lovely person took the time to meet with me on a regular basis. She and I focused first on our volunteer efforts but thankfully, as our friendship grew, we continued these monthly meetings. Without her realizing it, she began to mentor me. I felt comfortable asking her questions, simple advice. I realized right away that I could trust this friendship. That was important to me. As I grew, I also noticed the reciprocating of advice. We had come full circle in our mentor/friendship relationship. What a blessing that has been on so many levels of my life. When the Covid 19 pandemic struck, she and I committed to socially distance walking each week to stay healthy and accountable during that challenging time. And to mix things up, we even chose to pick different neighborhoods each week to walk around. Mentors mentoring each other.

So you see, networking does not need to be challenging, boring or monotonous. Take the time to connect and grow with outside groups as well as your healthcare world. The opportunities are endless and incredibly enriching. You can begin this process by volunteering in an area of your personal interest. Just go for it! I can't wait to see how many networking doors will open for you. However, it plays out, I hope you too can experience the boomerang effect networking blessings provide.

Reflection:

Spend some time identifying someone you would like to get to know more. Someone you admire. If this is a professional relationship, consider inviting this person out for lunch. If lunch doesn't work, consider taking a walk together. Maybe you'd rather attend a continuing education class together. Just begin at the beginning. Identify someone you admire and see if a mentoring relationship could blossom. Be gracious and grateful when receiving any advice from your mentor. And who knows, someone could reach out to you in the future and need your mentorship. It can truly be a beautiful circle of kindness and you are so worth it.

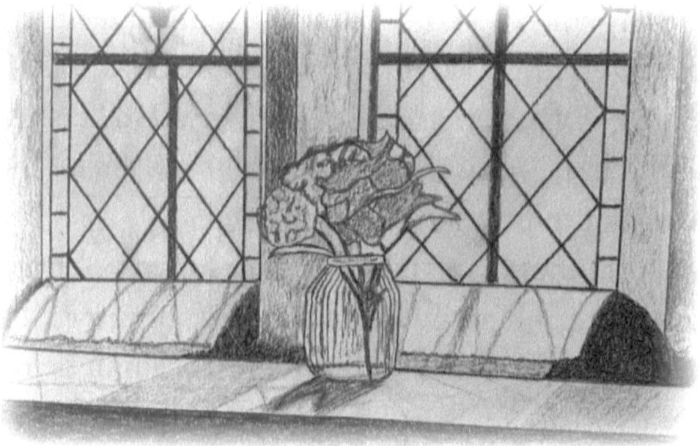

Mindful Living – Mindful Life

Chances are, that by now, you've noticed the essence of mindfulness sprinkled throughout these pages and in my life. Not sure if sprinkled is the right word though. You see, without the practice of mindfulness in my life, I'm not sure this book would even exist. For me, I need mindfulness slathered all over my life and in consistent doses, not just sprinklings. But again, that's just me. If you must know, my faith, family and heart-filled mindfulness are what I believe provided the fuel I needed to make this journey. And I love that! So true to my nature that mindful living would provide me with the clarity, stamina and energy needed to put my thoughts and experiences into written form. Mindfulness, not chaos, works for me. Although I have seen some amazing work come from creative chaos. It just doesn't work for me. So let me do a quick Mindfulness 101 for you.

Mindfulness. This word doesn't usually scream as a front-page headline. It's not the nature of mindfulness to jump out at you either. "Mindfulness is about being fully aware of whatever is happening in the present moment, without filters or the lens of judgment."[14] Today, I believe the practice of Mindfulness has the power and ability to affect all facets of our lives including our healthcare careers. In my mind and heart, I believe the practice of mindfulness has the potential to spill over into every nook and cranny of our personal and professional lives if invited. From complex clinical situations to learning how to safely move through a grocery store during a pandemic. Mindfulness can become a gentle fuel source for your soul. And it's free! Won't cost you a dime or be influenced by inflation either.

Just think about this for a moment. Pause and consider what it would be like to be so present with your healthcare patient or client, so attuned with your procedure that you

[14] Stahl, Bob PH.D, Goldstein, Elisha PH.D. *A Mindfulness-Based Stress Reduction Workbook*. New Harbinger Publications, Inc. 2010. Page 15

are alert yet not stressed, aware yet without judgment. In other words, finely tuned into the moment you are a part of. You may now be tempted to shout at me, "What if I don't want to be aware of my moment? I don't want to be fully present to the grumpy patient before me. I don't want to be tuned into another repetitive procedure that allows my mind to wander and causes my body to scream in pain." Let me first validate your feelings but also ask you to stay with me on this journey. You see, as the author of "What the Buddha Taught," Walpola Rahula states, "(Mindfulness) is simply observing, watching, examining. You are not a judge but a scientist."[15] Viewing every grumpy patient, every repetitive procedure, every challenge and success through the lens of a scientist could bring about a whole new perspective.

While practicing mindfulness you have the opportunity to become aware of new possibilities that your previously frustrated mind may have been blocking out. I liken it to the lifting of heaviness. It feels so liberating and accelerating to no longer live your life on auto pilot or tied up in frustration or judgment. When you leave the negativity of unhealthy thought patterns out of your mind, the world can and will change. There is so much light that can make its way into your soul with equal amounts flowing outward.

---

[15] Rahula, Walpola. *What the Buddha Taught.* New York. Grove Press. (1974)

Still interested in the science behind the practice of Mindfulness? Let's go a smidge deeper. Mindfulness addresses the physiological reaction your body has to stress. When you perceive a situation as a threat, the hypothalamus will prompt your adrenal glands to secrete cortisol and adrenalin. The release of adrenalin alone will cause elevated blood pressure and heart rates. Cortisol will then increase glucose in your bloodstream but it will also slow down other bodily functions. Basically, a stress storm is produced.

These physiological actions lead our bodies to choose between a fight, flight or freeze response. What the practice of Mindfulness attempts to do is teach a person to self-activate a different response to stress. Rather than staying in a state of heightened anxiety, fear, or soaring blood pressure, Mindfulness trains a person to kick in a formal or informal response to the stress. And for me, learning to bring mindfulness to the front of my brain instead of a stress response has changed my life. I use mindfulness skills all day long. From work to home life, I move in the world so much more thoughtfully when I use mindfulness skills. I feel calmer. More thoughtful. Less reactive. Hopefully, more loving. Do I do this perfectly? Heck no! Although I wish I lived in that mindfulness zone all the time, when I fall off the tracks, I am more quickly aware and able to return to the calm and clarity of mindfulness sooner.

So, if I still have your attention and willingness to stay open-minded, want to unpack this concept a little more?

I mentioned the words informal versus formal previously. Mindfulness is typically broken into a Formal versus Informal practice and it's actually quite simple. A Formal Mindfulness practice would be to *intentionally* take time out to meditate, Mindful walking,[16] practice Yoga, do a Mindfulness body scan[17] or even a Metta Meditation.[18] The keyword here is *intentional.* You plan and set aside time to do this.

An Informal Mindfulness practice requires a person to bring more attention to everyday tasks such as breathing, driving, walking, eating or any activity one does on a daily basis. For me, breathwork is the lifeline to a mindfulness zone. My breath helps me enter a mindful state of being, it also helps bring me back into mindfulness. Stress storms will happen in life. Guaranteed. They can slowly erupt or happen spontaneously. Today, however, I have tools that can provide me shelter from those storms. Formal or informal. Mindfulness works in my life.

Bottom line, whatever facet of the health profession you call home, I believe anyone can benefit from mindful living. Not just at work, but in all parts of your beautiful life. And what do you have to lose? Stress and chaos? Trust me, you won't miss those storms. So jump in. Consider taking a Mindfulness class or reading literature on

---

[16] http://www.mindfulnessatwork.ie/tips-for-mindful-walking/

[17] https://www.youtube.com/watch?v=SJxQ8CWxzPw

[18] http://www.mettainstitute.org/mettameditation.html

the topic. Lather yourself with mindfulness. Who knows, maybe a sprinkle or two of calmness and clarity will land on you and every person you connect with.

Reflection:

Do a quick google search on the practice of mindfulness. Just go out there and look around. See if you might be interested in exploring this practice. Maybe you'd like to take a Mindfulness class or consider downloading a Mindfulness app on your phone. If this puts too much pressure on you. Let it go. If it is meant for you, it will happen when it is supposed to. And remember, you are worth it!

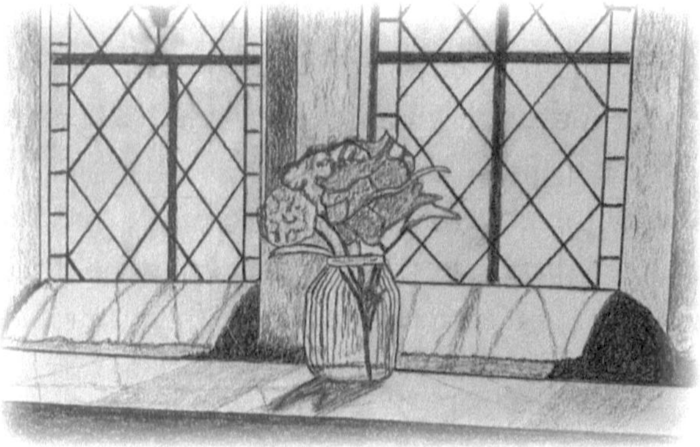

Why We Do What We Do

If you circle back to the beginning of this book you may recall me prompting you to reach back and discover why you entered the healthcare profession. What were your motivational forces? Were they financial, inspirational and/or circumstantial? Did passion exist in your decision-making process, had it seeped into your already established career or were you still uncovering it? Well, it wasn't until I stumbled across Simon Sinek's TED Talk, "How Great Leaders Inspire Actions"[19] that I realized how critical the

[19] https://www.ted.com/talks/simon_sinek_how_great_leaders_inspire_action

foundational "why" questions really were. Without even knowing it, I had begun at the beginning. Exactly where Simon would have encouraged me to start. "People don't buy what you do, they buy why you do it." Big difference. Let's break it apart.

Simon Sinek, author and inspirational speaker, first reached my heart after listening to his 2014 TED Talk, "How Great Leaders Inspire Actions." In my humble opinion, his work is brilliant. Simply brilliant. In fact, I revisit Simon's Ted talk at least annually. His talk is so down to earth and it really helped polish some of my career skills and daily actions. If you've got time, why not check it out? Scoop up some of Simon's wisdom. If you don't have time, the following is what I've gleaned from his Ted Talk.

Starting at the beginning, Simon encourages everyone to consider "Why" you do what you do. Simon boldly states "People don't buy what you do, they buy why you do it." It's that simple. Why do you do what you do? He sites that many corporations and individuals know **wha**t they do and **how** they do it, they just neglect to define **why** they do what they do. Simon illustrated this beautifully with his "Golden Circle" concept.

Simon mentions several times that many great companies, such as Apple and great speakers, such as Dr. Martin Luther King Jr., moved through the world differently than most of us. They seemed to act from the inside out. They always started with the why and then moved to the what and how. That concept seemed so foreign to me but I was intrigued. I knew I needed to apply his wisdom to my own world. Simply put, I needed to begin answering the What, How and Why questions in my own life to see how it would play out. Did I work from the outside in or the opposite?

So here's what I discovered. Before listening to Simon Sinek's talk, I typically answered questions in this manner and order:

> **What**: I am a Registered Dental Hygienist.
>
> **How**: Within the educational framework of my Dental Hygiene license, I provide compassionate, high level, thorough, up to date, dental hygiene services to every patient I serve.
>
> **Why** I want to journey alongside every dental patient I serve by offering them excellent, thorough and encouraging dental hygiene care. I want to individualize my treatment towards them. I want to assure each patient they are not alone, they are safe and they matter to me!

After I mindfully reviewed Simon's talk, I attempted to answer the "Why" questions first. I wanted to just check out the Golden Circle process to see if it looked or felt any different. Below are the same words I used in the above statements, they are just ordered differently. Check it out.

> **Why**: I want to journey alongside every dental patient I serve by offering them excellent, thorough and encouraging dental hygiene care. I want to individualize my treatment towards them. I want to assure each patient they are not alone, they are safe and they matter to me!
>
> **How**: Within the educational framework of my Dental Hygiene license, I provide compassionate, high level, thorough, up to date, dental hygiene services to every patient I serve.
>
> **What**: I am a Registered Dental Hygienist.

What are your thoughts? If you read my professional bio on a website which order of information would you like to see me lead off with? What would get your attention? I personally would rather know why someone or a business does what they do before I dig into the details. Don't get me wrong. I want the details. They are critical. It's just when you lead with the why question first, you've got my attention until the end. That's just how my brain works. So why not give this a try. Have some fun with it. See where the Golden Circle takes you. If you're not ready to dig into your professional goals and dreams begin with your personal life. Trust me, there's a golden circle waiting for you to uncover. Go for it! Jump in and watch how far the ripples go.

Reflection:

Carve out some quiet time to reflect on the question, why you do what you do. Decide if you want to focus on your personal or professional life. After answering the why question, circle back around to the how and what questions. Collect your discoveries and find a way to make this information visible to you. Find a space to help you remember the whys, especially on the days when the what and hows are overtaking your life. Remember, you're worth it!

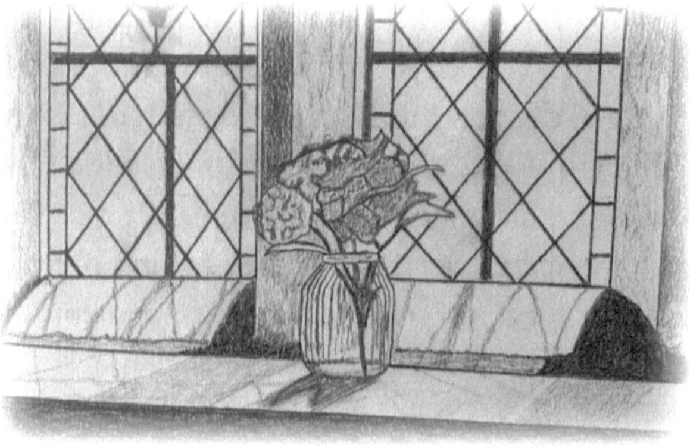

Under the Radar

Playing it safe can feel good. I won't lie, most of my life, I've played it safe. I lacked the confidence in myself to really become who I was purposed to be. To take risks. To succeed. To fail. Basically, to live as an imperfect human being. For me, this behavior defect played out in my professional life too. For too long I stayed quiet when I should have spoken up at staff meetings or communicated more truthfully with co-workers. I lived under the radar instead of in the light.

I think for me, I let my people-pleasing chromosomes keep me under the radar of life, both personally and professionally. Looking back, I bet I drove a few people crazy living this way. I suspect they were easily frustrated with me when I lacked the confidence to voice my opinions or even make concise decisions. I never set out to live this way though. What, at one time, was probably a beneficial life skill eventually morphed into a character challenge. I knew I wanted to change. I wanted to find my voice, so I began to focus on my personal development and not everyone else around me. Game changer!

How did I tackle this challenge? As I previously mentioned, I started connecting weekly with someone I deeply admired. Someone I had gotten to know while serving on a nonprofit organization. We were just two volunteers with very different backgrounds. We first began meeting when trying to help organize a fundraising event. Little by little as we met, I started to glean personal confidence that seemed to spill out professionally as well. Thankfully, when I approached this person and asked if she would consider mentoring me, meeting with me monthly, offering me guidance, she accepted. It was at that moment two things happened. I was no longer on my own island of isolation and secondly, I felt hope in my personal development. And hope, my friends, is priceless! For me, having hope helped me see the world with a wider lens. Having someone to mentor me, join me on my radar screen of life was a life-changing decision. For me, it has become a wonderful, trusting friendship as well as mentorship. In fact, without my mentor's encouragement to continue writing, I doubt I would be where I am today. Or at least, it would have taken me much longer to arrive.

Let me get a little honest with you right now. The behaviors that started changing, that helped me find my way onto the radar screen of life, were very subtle changes. They didn't happen overnight but they were so worth it. When my mentor shared how she handled a work situation, I began to notice how she mentally stayed connected to the issue but was better able to emotionally detach from the situation than I was. Her approach was still very heartfelt, it was just not all heart-consuming. She didn't dwell on the situation for days. She knew how to handle it and then let it go. So, little by little I began to apply those simple skills to patient and co-worker interactions as well. I began to notice how emotionally invested I would be in an interchange, sometimes for days. I would allow my brain to overthink, to vacillate about the situation. After watching my mentor handle similar interactions, I realized it was a learned skill that allowed her to emotionally detach without losing the personal connection she was vested in. Oh, did I want to sign up for that class. Thought I'd call it, Healthy Detachment 101.

There was something else I began to notice. My mentor handled failure, or in her world, "learning experiences" very differently than I did. I watched her share experiences that did not have desired outcomes. I would then listen to her work through those situations. She always came out with a learning experience to take away, to learn from.

Right there, my friends, was my golden ticket to leaping onto the radar screen of my life. My mentor knew how and when to learn from the situation and then to let it go. She had trained her brain to not see failure but to instead see learning opportunities. She was able to move on, to stay on that radar screen of life instead of hiding in the darkness. For me, learning this skill has taken years. Detaching and letting go of failure is not easy for me but doing so is so liberating.

Another priceless nugget of learning my mentor shared was how to recognize your part of the learning situation. To help me gently discover what was my part of the learning opportunity. To then learn how to correct it, if necessary. To forgive myself and/or the other person involved. To learn how to make an appropriate amend. This is so important. Staying authentic on the radar screen of life may require some uncomfortable actions from you. Forgiving others is not always easy, forgiving yourself, sometimes even harder. Offering a heartfelt apology is actually one of the healthiest skills you will ever learn though. A life skill that will help you continue living your best life. Not a perfect life. Something even better. Your best life. No longer do you have to carry the weight of guilt, shame or an unforgiving heart. You just have to be willing to show up, learn from the situation, change your behavior if necessary and make an amend if needed. You can be fully present on life's radar screen, not just a soft blimp in the background.

What might happen if you are willing to try living this way? To learn heartfelt detachment. To learn how to make mistakes, make amends and then to let go. Well, my friend, prepare to light up your radar screen. If you are like me, you'll notice more comfort in approaching others when you have concerns. You'll notice you may begin to enjoy finding your voice in office-staff meetings. Your personal life may also light up too. It's a simple formula but has tremendous potential to create authentic changes in your life. And who says life has to be complicated? I continue to watch my mentor move through many challenging life circumstances without getting bogged down. I can only hope and pray I've learned to do the same. And who knows, maybe we'll light the way for others to find their true selves.

Sound too Utopian? Heaven on earth? Bliss? Nirvana? Call it what you like, but today, I truly believe we can all work towards living and working more fully in the light. We can work towards creating a culture that accepts and allows everyone to be more fully human. To succeed, to make errors, to learn, to grow, to live fully on the radar screen of life. Might take a little self-retrospection to jump back on the grid but I promise you it will be worth it. Consider taking this journey with a friend, a mentor or even a therapist. Someone you trust. Someone you can begin to uncover your stuff with and what is keeping you from living a fuller life. I can't promise you this journey will be a sprint. Rather, it may look more like a marathon.

But that's ok. There is no time limit to arriving on the grid, to discovering your true self, to learn how to take risks that will lead you to a more authentic life. And who knows, maybe someday you'll be blessed to join someone else on their radar screen of life. Become a mentor, friend, a confidant. That, my friend, is when your light will truly shine. What are you waiting for? Our world longs to meet you, the real you.

Reflection:

I think it might be time to have a little fun. To fill up our life buckets with joy in order to be more fully present on life's radar screen. What do you like to do that brings you joy? Do you like to bike ride? Visit the library? Connect with a friend? Build a snowman outside? How about building a sandcastle? What about hunkering down to watch a movie? Decide what brings you joy and jump in. Have some fun. Bring your whole self to life and begin lighting up your radar screen. We need that light, and you are so worth it!

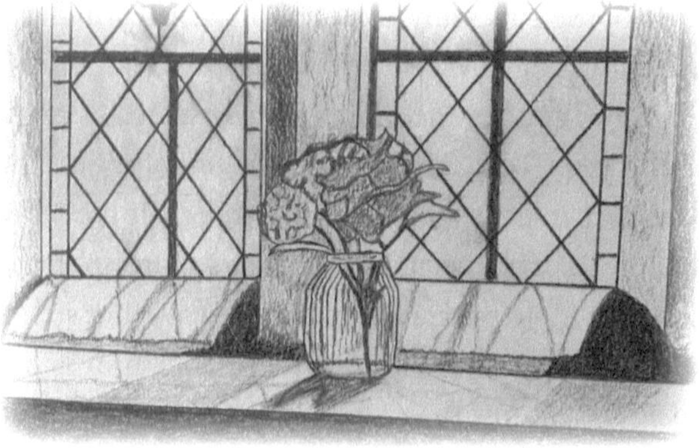

I Know and Remember Your Name

I hope we've all experienced, at least once in our career, a moment of pure joy and satisfaction when a healthy behavior or improved health condition is established. For me, those moments are magnified whenever I am working with a patient with differing emotional, mental and/or physical needs. Mind you, in one way or another, I believe we all live life differently. We each have a special way of learning, physically moving and expressing ourselves. In our own way, we are each special and gifted and deserving of respect for our uniqueness. But what if that uniqueness caused you hardship? What if you moved in this world outside of the culturally accepted norms? If you did, could you just imagine how far a few simple acts of kindness could go in your life? Let me offer you a few ideas I've gleaned over the years that have helped me show more kindness and respect to every patient, co-worker, employer, family and friend I have been privileged to share space on this earth with. A few ideas that I hope have blessed others. Ideas I know that have blessed me!

The first thing that pops into my mind and heart is how we identify each other. How we greet each other or refer to each other. I believe there is a sacred connection established when you use someone's name. That's right. Using someone's name in conversation with them. In my humble opinion, when someone speaks your name with kindness, it can lead to a gentler space of communication and trust. Think about it. Are you more likely to tune into someone who uses your name and not a derogatory nick-name or limp pronoun? Think about those we serve in the healthcare profession. I personally think that politely using someone's name is a simple show of respect but sadly I've seen its usage waiver. Maybe not purposely, but I've noticed it happening more and more. In-person and even on social media platforms. Let's try and change that.

Well, as the world blessed me unexpectedly a few years back I had some wonderful disability training that highlighted the use of "People First Language." Even mentioning this training may seem trite but stay with me. Person First Language is not trite. I believe this is too important to overlook. Trust me, this could be such a game-changer in your professional and personal life.

People First Language[20] puts the emphasis on the person and not their differences. It is as simple as using phrases such as "Susie, my college roommate. Johnny, my beloved patient with Downs Syndrome. Mary, my friend who struggles with anxiety. Eleanor, my next-door neighbor." Everyone is a person first. A person with a name. Please begin your communication with that sign of respect. Make it a point for you to learn their name and to pronounce it correctly too. I've even had to make several phonetic notes on patient charts that help me pronounce names correctly. And when I'm in doubt, I politely ask the patient to correct or affirm my pronunciation. Even doing that can express a genuine act of kindness.

After you commit this person's name to your mind and heart it might direct you to educate yourself in order to better accommodate your patient's needs. Do a little homework friend. I believe this is critical. Will you be working with someone who displays Autism Spectrum Disorder behaviors? Consider sending a visual flow chart to their home before their first appointment. This could easily be a collection of pictures, all copied onto an 8X11 piece of paper. Pictures that include who the patient will

[20] https://www.verywellfamily.com/focus-on-the-person-first-is-good-etiquette-2161897

be working with, what your waiting room looks like, what the clinician room looks like, what the healthcare provider looks like in full gear. Photos of anything you think might help your patient adjust to your surroundings more easily. Have this done ahead of time so you can mail it to your patient before their first appointment. This will help prepare your patient before they even arrive in the office.

I also advise practitioners to look at their work space in order to evaluate lighting issues. If bright lights are too stimulating, have sunglasses ready and available for your patient. What about noise issues, excessive audio stimulation? Noise-canceling headphones are a possible solution to that challenge. Gentle background music can also help create a more comfortable environment for your patient. Introduce instruments and other adjuncts slowly and cautiously. Taking the time to establish and record specific routines your patient exhibits during your appointment will allow you the opportunity to continue building a healthy relationship. You may want to also note concerns. Whatever comes up during this appointment, discuss everything with their family member and/or staff. Some of your greatest career satisfaction moments may come from these precious experiences.

What if your friend or family member uses a walker or wheelchair to move through the world? Making sure your waiting room, restroom and patient care room are all wheelchair accessible is the minimum we must all achieve. Do your best to physically match their line of vision as well. I find this so overlooked but such a huge courtesy. Make sure, when you can, to sit down and face your patient. It may seem like a simple, unnecessary thing to do, but just put yourself in their wheelchair. Would you like to have to always crank your neck upward to see who is talking to you? And always make sure you ask permission before you help your patient move their wheelchair. Keep in mind, their wheelchair is an extension of their own bodies. Seek permission first. I also personally like to add extra time to my schedule when working with mobility differences.

I think it is also worth noting that by law, every business must accommodate for those accessibility issues. Can you transfer these adjustments to help create barrier-free movement in your home. Why not consider installing a portable ramp in your home if a friend or family needs that assistance? I regret I didn't make that happen when my parents and in-laws were aging. We were always able to help them move in and out of our home, but it could have been much easier. And what a visible sign of love and respect that could have been. One thing we did try to do was to remove small rugs in our home. Seeking this advice from an Occupational Therapist definitely reinforced how rugs can easily become tripping hazards. We were also able to adapt our bathrooms to help with that aspect of life.

There are so many portals to obtain barrier-free devices and information, whether you are searching online or can visit a Home Health Care Supply store in person. You won't regret taking the time to do this. There are so many pearls of information and acts of kindness just waiting for you to scoop up. Don't hesitate to share what you uncover with your team members or family members. Just take a moment, pause, and get to know someone's name.

Reflection:

How would you like someone to introduce you? What adjectives and adverbs would you want used to describe you? Spend some time thinking about this and then write it down. Make sure you put your name first. And who knows, it just might inspire you. Never forget, you're worth it and so is everyone else on this planet.

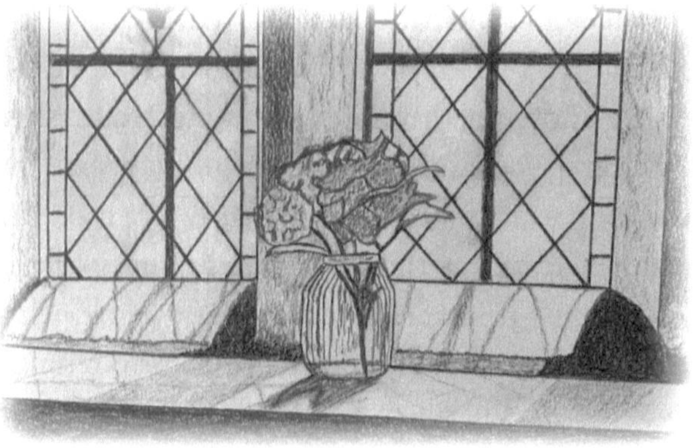

It's Hard to Be Me Without You

It's hard to be me without you. I blurted the previous statement out to my co-worker one morning after having to temporarily work in a more isolated area the previous day. I simply stated, "it's hard to be me, without you." This person looked at me with the simple recognition of that statement. They got it. It's not that either one of us couldn't function on our own, it's just we were sharper, more ourselves when we were connected to each other in our work environment. We, together, created a comfortable, supportive working environment.

Quite simply, we always wanted the best for each other, our families and the patients we served.

If you are presently working in that type of environment you know exactly what I am talking about. #Priceless. Do whatever you can to continue fostering that environment. Support each other, forgive each other. Be there for each other. If that is the environment you work in, you know it is just priceless. You are able to signal when you need help running your work schedule or commitments. How about needing help when you are running behind. Do you work with people that are willing to help get you back on track? Are you willing to help others catch back up as well? I've personally been so blessed when other co-workers have offered to help me if they had time to do so. Sometimes their schedule is derailed too. When that happens, I personally feel humbled to help others that need any assistance. Sometimes all I can do is pray for my coworker though, but I believe that is priceless too.

In my opinion, kindness crosses over any department. Kindness can flow anywhere. When you have free time, asking the front desk team members if you can help them is a genuine act of kindness. You may not have all the skills and training to help in all ways, but I imagine you could at least help refile patient charts. And in my opinion. A team member does not leave for the day until they have asked all remaining co-workers how they can help finish their day. Just a simple "How can I help" before you leave the building goes a long way. And it's so simple! Nine times out of ten team members tell me they are all set, but every so often someone will have a very simple task for me to do. What a blessing to be able to help someone in need and what a beautiful way to continue fostering healthy relationships.

If you aren't fortunate enough to work in that type of environment ask yourself a few questions. Is there something you could do to improve the situation? Keep in mind, there is usually no quick fix and I also believe everyone holds a piece of the truth. A solution may take time but it could be worth the wait. Maybe the situation calls for a third party to assist you. An office manager could really help resolve some of your differences and set you all on a different track. This may take a leap of faith and an element of trust but again could be priceless in changing your working atmosphere. Another possible game-changer in working environments is to attend a dental conference together. Consider going out to lunch together. Getting out of the office can sometimes open up time and opportunities to better understand each other's lives. Many people today carry heavy burdens they try to keep from spilling out into their work lives. You may be able to help shoulder their burdens, maybe not. But at a minimum, you will obtain a better understanding of each other.

If, after all possible adjustments and effort are tried, you are still not comfortable in your work environment you may need to plan an exit strategy. If this is the only option left before you, I urge you to keep this in mind. Parting ways doesn't have to be anyone's fault. It doesn't make you right or wrong. It doesn't make your co-worker right or wrong. It could just be a matter of incompatibility. You just have to decide if you can work in that type of environment or need to seek employment elsewhere. Remember, in life, not everything needs to be labeled as success or failure. It's all just learning. And that, my friend, is a beautiful way to live.

Reflection:

Take some time to reflect on your working and personal relationships. Are you someone who easily offers to help others in need? Note I am not suggesting you enable others to neglect their duties on a regular basis. I am just asking you to create some safe space to evaluate how you support others in your life. This may take some time to really uncover. Don't rush the process. You might even consider journaling what you discover. Whatever comes up, it will be a blessing and a wonderful guidepost. Never forget you are worth it!

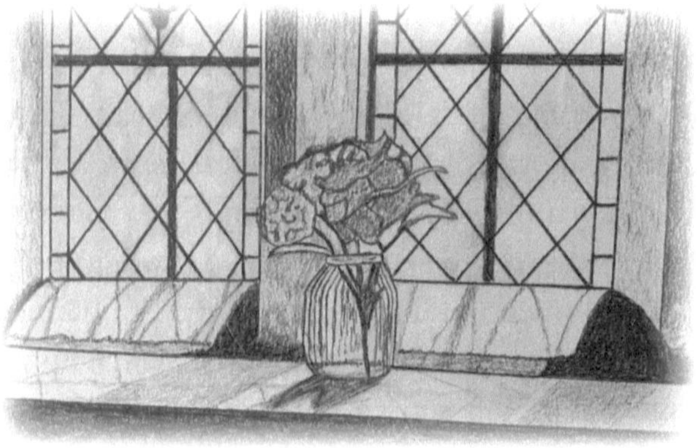

What Do You Geek?

In 2009, the Bill and Melinda Gates Foundation launched the "What do you geek?" campaign aimed at bringing awareness to our public libraries. I happened to be at a high school football game when I first stumbled upon this effort. And as I reflect back on that moment, it was all serendipity. A cool, crisp fall evening. A high school football team charging a grassy field. Fans huddled together on the bleachers. The high school band playing in the background. Lots of energy and people swirling all around. Just a perfect night for sipping some concession stand hot chocolate and eating some buttered popcorn.

True to my nature, I set out to purchase some popcorn, chocolate-covered peanut candy and, of course, my customary cup of cocoa. I then headed back to my seat in the bleachers. Right at this time though, I also noticed a crowd of people gathering near the stadium fence line. Turns out, our local library had hitched a ride on the "What do you Geek?" train and was gaining some positive momentum during this football gathering. With chalkboard in hand, these volunteers were simply asking people, "What do you geek?" A person would then use chalk to write on this board what they geeked. Someone took your picture and then posted those photos onto the library's website. It was just a blast! How could I resist this chance to express my geekiness, so I dove in.

When my turn in line finally arrived, I picked up some chalk and proudly shared a piece of my zealous geeky nature. Without hesitation, I scrolled "I Geek a Smile." A smile. A simple smile. And we, my friends, and professional comrades are blessed to be a part of bringing smiles to life. I can personally testify what it's like to hide your smile, be ashamed of your smile, to constantly bring your hand to your mouth when you smile. It's exhausting. It's also been heartbreaking to live behind our much-needed masks during the Covid 19 Pandemic. Did you miss seeing smiles too? I know I sure did.

So why don't we get a little geeky about helping others bring their smiles to life? Let's recharge and remind each other what some of our core principles in our healthcare fields are. Trust me on this, whatever tangent of the healthcare field you are in, you can influence anyone's smile. You can help provide and even restore confidence in someone's ability to smile. To me, a smile radiates and communicates so much. When someone smiles, whatever the age, you need to engage both your inner soul as well as physical musculature. It's an inside and outside job to smile genuinely.

So let's get geeky and try to uncover what brings some joy to professional life first. What do you geek professionally? What brings a smile to your face when you think about your career? Is it achieving, maintaining and/or improving your patient's optimal health? Attending continuing education classes? Seriously, what most excites you about your healthcare career? For me, I most definitely geek "connections" in my professional life. Not surprising to anyone who knows me that I look for connections everywhere. Connections with my patients and my co-workers. When a connection is established I feel more empowered to be my "geeky" best. When I've connected to my patient's needs, my internal filing systems take off and begin to formulate a suggested treatment plan, home care regimen, continuing care needs or even a restorative sequence they may need to follow. But that's how my brain ticks. I dare you to uncover what you geek most in your career. What gets you excited to come to work? What gives you the drive to perform your best while working into your lunch hour? Think about it, then geek about it.

Write it down. Post it somewhere so you can be reminded where your career passions lie.

Still feeling brave? Let's take a walk, or tip toe, into your personal world. What about your private life do you geek? Would it be family, music, yoga, running marathons, meditation, scrapbooking, reading to your grandchildren, volunteering, playing racquetball, knitting, painting with watercolors, boating, gardening, writing, snowboarding, walking outside? Does this list seem endless to you? In truth, the list could very well be infinite. It also seems sprinkled with many more "fun" activities rather than work-related. Deep down, I really hope your personal geeky list does fill up faster than your professional list. If it doesn't that's ok too. We all need to start somewhere. Just remember, forward is forward, no matter the speed.

Who knows? Maybe we all desire to exist in our personal world a little more than our professional. Or, maybe it's actually quite balanced. Maybe it's not balanced. Could it be that our personal geeky stuff crosses over into our professional world every so often though? I have found that my love for walking outdoors lives in both my professional and personal worlds. I love days that I have enough time to walk outside during my lunch hour. I also love prayer and meditation which easily lives in both my professional and personal spaces. For me, the merger of my geekiness is when I am my most authentic and vulnerable self. When those moments happen, it's beautiful.

Truth is, I really do “Geek a smile.” I geek smiles at work. I geek smiles everywhere. A quote by Max Beerbohm states, “I need no dictionary of quotations to remind me that the eyes are the window of the soul.”[21] Well, it’s my belief that every human can actually see into one’s soul through a smile. So whether you share it, help create it or nurture it. I dare you to get geeky about smiles! It’s the wheelhouse I live and work in and I love it!

Reflection:

What do you geek? Write it down. Draw it out and then take a selfie. Find a way to post what you geek and then, get geeky about it!

[21] http://thinkexist.com/quotation/i_need_no_dictionary_of_quotations_to_remind_me/196883.html

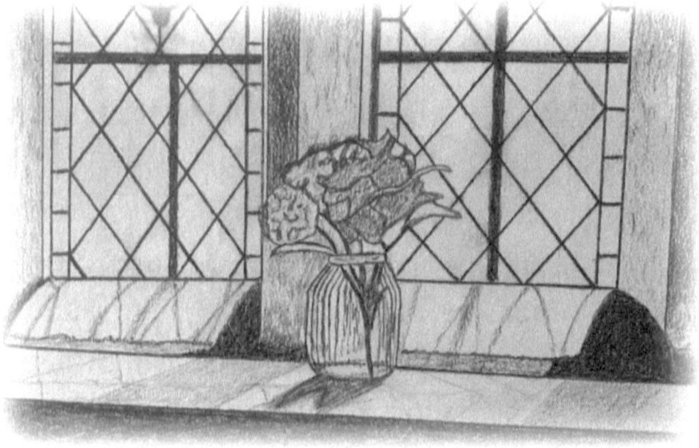

Circle Time

I would love to know if you have any memories of preschool circle time? Is this ringing any school bells? Maybe the connections are from your own children's experience of circle time. If you are closer to my age, circle time may not have been available to you in preschool though. For me, my first memories of school are all contained in a small kindergarten classroom. Any chance you could take yourself back and visualize one of those sweet rooms, filled with colorful toys, squares of carpet, child-sized chairs and tables, wonderful books, colorful crayons, maybe some markers and if you are lucky, maybe some finger paints. If I pause long enough I swear I can still smell that finger paint. I can even hear the energetic buzz of young children moving around the room. Did you have a cubby to store your things in? Maybe a hook for your jacket?

Before I get lost going down memory lane and believe me I could, let's circle back to circle time. Any chance you have a memory of the gathering rug found almost universally in those sweet classrooms? The gathering rug, where circle time happened. Do you remember this rug? If not in your early educational experience it might have been there for your son or daughter's experience. Some of those precious rugs were designed with animals around their circumferences. Some had alphabet letters or creative numbers all brilliantly designed and spaced for young children to sit around.

At first glance, those early childhood gathering rugs may not seem like an important item to discuss, but I believe they truly are. Think about it. This is where children begin to learn how to gather as a community. It is where they learn to listen to each other's ideas and comments. It's where they find their voice as well as their listening ears. It's where they come to rest, to sit by a friend or even sit next to a stranger. It's where the expression of community can begin to happen and it's right there on a simple rug.

I have such a soft spot in my heart for early childhood educators and their programs. I only wish all those early life lessons could be permanently imprinted on every human's heart and mind. Sadly, I think, life has a way of erasing those precious learning moments. Some days it's just hard to remember to bring our circle time behavior to work with us. I know there are days when I slip into ego-driven behavior instead of loving my neighbor. Not proud of those moments. Thankful I can catch myself and work through some strategies that can swing me back to a healthier way of moving in the world. It will always be my hope that every classroom in life would still be able to reinforce those preschool skills, those precious values. The ability to sit together in a circle, share your thoughts, listen to others, be next to a friend or a stranger.

I genuinely believe these circle time spaces exist in our healthcare work environments. I have personally worked with a group of professionals who gather each morning for a team huddle. No, we don't get to sit down on a rug and share snacks but we do get to share thoughts and concerns for the day. It's a chance for our team to communicate the game plan for the day, at least how we hope it will play out. Sometimes this space has allowed staff members the opportunity to share very joyful news but it is also a space that heartbreaking news can be shared as well. I believe, creating a dedicated "circle time" in your office can help strengthen office communication as well. The information doesn't need to be shared over and over again. The information can be shared during the huddle, everyone hears it from the same person and can then move on much easier. In my opinion, this time is priceless!

What about the other spaces in our lives where circle time can happen? Spaces and moments where your personal and family values can be shared, respected and hopefully retained. Do you gather anywhere in particular as a family? Around the dining room table or kitchen island? Is there a space in your own home that your family knows they can come to, be accepted and listened to? Personally, we always shared our evening meal around the kitchen table. We attempted to create a safe and welcoming space for our family. Not sure that always happened with four children, but that was always our prayer. I've also heard from other friends that their car became a special place where conversation flowed, where opinions were respected and listened to. Your gathering space need never be on a rug or at the kitchen table. Just be creative when cultivating your family's circle time atmosphere. This treasured space could really open up, add to and even restore relationships.

What about outside your work or family unit? Try not to laugh, but every time I enter an exercise room and then find my space on the floor, it also reminds me of circle time. Think about it. We're all gathering, sharing space with others. We're all there, gathered in that space for a common cause. To sweat a little, burn off some calories, release some stress and hopefully become a better version of ourselves.

I've also witnessed a beautiful circular flow of kindness in some volunteer organizations I've been a part of. How about you? I've seen it happen over and over again when you hope to be the one "giving" and you then find yourself "receiving." It's the space I long to exist in, whether I'm home, at work or volunteering in the community.

If for any reason you find yourself in situations that lack core preschool values let me validate that you are not alone. It does happen and it's not easy to navigate life when it takes you off the circle time gathering rug. Whether you are at home, at work or in the community, I encourage you to hold fast to your values of integrity. You don't have to go off-road. You can stay on the circle time rug or even bring your healthy values to another gathering rug. You can sit next to anyone and let them talk while you listen. I dare you to see if you can still sit criss-cross applesauce. Go for it! Run joyfully into the gathering spaces of life. They're really not that scary.

Reflection:

Where are the circle time spaces in your life? Can you identify an area in your home life that you would like to protect or possibly build upon? What about your professional life. Do you have space when your team gathers? Is it daily? Monthly? Maybe carving out that professional space won't be possible for you to do. You could consider helping create a newsletter at work. Not a gossip-filled newsletter. Rather something simple and filled with needed information. Go for it! Jump into those circle time spaces of life. And remember, you are worth it!

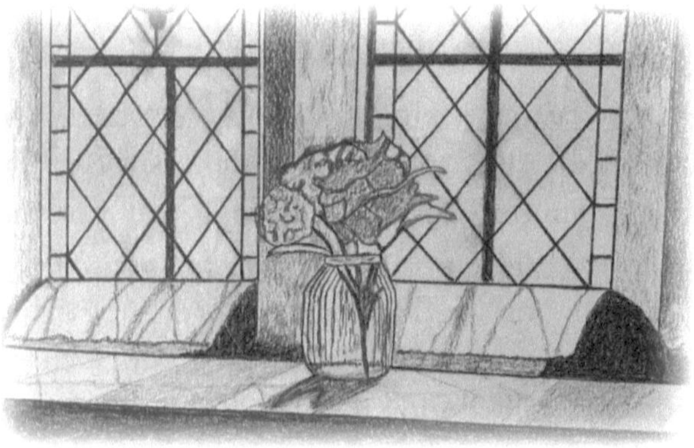

Trickle Down

The late 2000s held a significant financial marker in our nation's history and in many of our lives. I for one "thought" I was on track to retire in my early 50's. My husband and I had lived modestly, saved appropriately and were anticipating helping all four of our daughters receive a college education. The Great Recession had other plans for us though. Jump ahead to 2020 where the world experienced wildfire infections caused by the Coronavirus Pandemic. Again, we were all taken by surprise and thrown into many significant physical, mental and financial challenges. As I reflect on those moments in time, I realize how fortunate my family was and still is. Does this mean we haven't endured hardships? Absolutely not. We have and probably will still battle significant challenges. What seems to be our saving grace? Our attitude, the only thing we ever had control of in the first place. As soon as we committed ourselves to living and working with gratefulness and not bitterness, of looking outward and not inward, our world and our hearts opened right up.

And what a saving grace those values were for our family, especially during the Covid 19 pandemic. I wonder, with great humility, if your family or healthcare profession was impacted by this global situation? If by chance you have no memory of these events, allow me to trickle down a quick snapshot of what many of our healthcare providers went through.

For some of us, our healthcare offices were ordered to close temporarily. We were allowed to provide emergency care only. What we hoped would be only a few weeks, turned into months for some, depending on where you lived. In theory, this could be interpreted as a mini-vacation but trust me, it wasn't. To experience an abrupt change in your work habits and routines, to realize your absence was putting your patients at risk, to wonder how long or if you'll be allowed to return to work was all very uncomfortable.

I have to be honest, although what I experienced was uncomfortable, in my humble opinion, it was nothing compared to what our frontline healthcare workers who worked tirelessly throughout the pandemic had to confront. These courageous healthcare professionals continued to serve others while putting themselves at great risk day after day, shift after shift. They bravely had to work through the challenges of PPE shortages coupled with rising fears. These brave humans redefined what heroes really look like. I pray a steady trickle downstream of gratitude to each and every one of these brave humans.

I truly believe that the trickle-down effect of this health crisis and any other future challenges always has the potential to spill out trials and treasure. And in my opinion, it all comes down to your attitude. How you frame your situation will help determine what trickles out of you. The financial, emotional and mental challenges we all personally and professionally endured were significant and could take years to fully unpack. Moving through those situations was not easy and probably will never be easy. But if you are willing to work through them, the blessings could trickle down for a lifetime. When I look back at that moment in time, I credit our dental practice's ability to recover to the doctor who led us through with wisdom, compassion and great communication skills. He was able to project information as well as empathy for all staff members. Those actions inspired me to continue co-leading, with my husband, our family through that pandemic with similar attributes. I tell you, trickling down the good stuff is a beautiful thing!

Today I choose to focus on what I've been blessed with, no matter how small. For me, it has been so humbling to see what my time, talent and sometimes pennies can make a difference in our world. And I love thinking about the trickle-down effect those actions could have. What about you, both personally and professionally? If you're in a rut, first of all, you are not alone. What can you do though to give back to the world around you? Visit a neighbor, serve a meal at a local soup kitchen, mentor a youth, coach an athletic team, visit assisted living homes or send a card of encouragement to someone struggling.

What about your professional life? Consider sending notes of encouragement to your patients. What about checking in on a co-worker who is not feeling well? You could also volunteer at your affiliated healthcare clinics. Why not lead an effort to spruce up your office's outdoor landscaping? Add some potted flowers. Try to create a more inviting waiting area for your patients and even coworkers.

I realize this list is endless and that is actually exciting to me. You see, I believe that when we all show up to the party, it's where love grows. It's where kindness, compassion and generosity are born. It's what battles fear, anxiety and isolation. And our world needs you, it needs all of us. Maybe you even need to put yourself on that list? Just remember, the thief of joy is comparison so don't compare your actions to anyone else. Know what is in your heart and believe what you share can trickle down into the world around us. It does make a difference, one drop of kindness at a time.

Reflection:

Wherever you are in your life, I challenge you to bring to mind a life experience you could reframe. A new way of looking at a situation that could allow treasures to trickle out of you instead of continued trials? Spend some quiet time reflecting on the word "reframe." See where it leads you. See if you could either unplug a portal of kindness or create a new trickle downstream of it. Remember, that stream may need to circle around your heart for a while before it flows outward. And that's okay because you are so worth it.

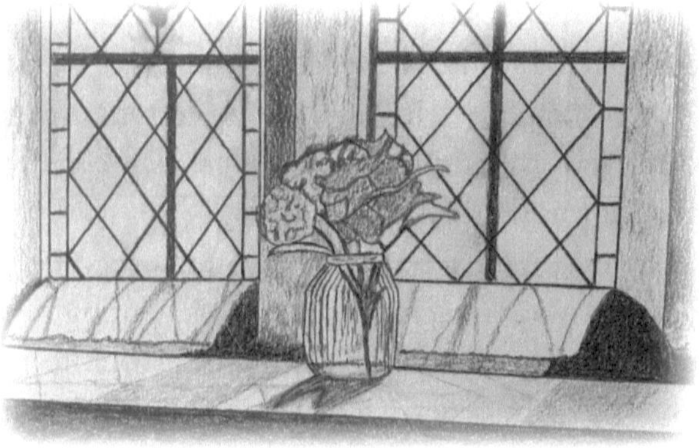

Consider It All Pure Joy

I knew this was going to be the hardest chapter for me to write. I just knew it! If you've come this far with me, you've probably already figured out that I'm an "all-in kind of human." Seems like everything I do, I put my whole self into it. So, no surprise it would be hard for me to even think about retiring from my beloved career. You see, my dental career truly has been pure joy. Notice I didn't say, all joy. I said pure joy. It wasn't until my cancer diagnosis that I allowed myself the space to pause, reflect and recognize what my career really meant to me though. I allowed myself the time to remember the many bumpy roads I had traveled. The smooth expressways too. The mistakes I'd made, the blessings I've received, the challenges I've encountered and the challenges I overcame. I was finally able to make peace with all of it, be enormously grateful and to view everything as joy. Join me as I share how I arrived at this destination.

For me, it first began with embracing that "I was enough." I was enough whether I was wearing my RDH hat, my family hat or my community volunteer hat or no hat! Deeply believing that personal statement freed up space in me to move forward on this journey towards retirement.

The next space I needed to evaluate was my physical condition. Was I strong enough to remain in, or return to, my beloved career? When and if I did, would I have the same stamina I once had? This may be a question for you to ask yourself and you don't need to wait until there is a medical challenge. For me, I didn't know the answers to those questions until I attempted to return to work, which I eventually did. I am grateful to share that I was able to return to my career and feel great! If your physical condition is showing you that retirement or career change is in your near future, I truly believe another door or window will open for you.

Emotional health and stability. Is your whole heart still in the game? I decided, based on the way I am wired, that I needed to address this question early on. Personally, I give my whole heart to whatever I'm doing. Now, that is not always the healthy thing to do, it's just the way I'm made. So, no surprise that my emotional health needed to be evaluated. What about yours? Are you still emotionally in the game? Can you still hold each patient you serve with kindness and compassion? If not, this could be an indicator that you need to step away from your career. Again, trusting another window or door will open for you.

Mental health. Are you making mental mistakes? Are you still mentally present when you step foot into your healthcare office? I personally attempt to give my best every day but can also share that when I'm dealing with enormous stress, it is a challenge to stay mentally attuned. If you are feeling mentally drained, yet want to remain in your career, see what other factors may be attributed to that situation. Consult a doctor. Talk to a friend. See if you need to adapt your lifestyle in order to keep you mentally sharp and as effective as possible. Are you attending Continuing Education classes? Are you still seeking new information relevant to your profession? If you've stopped doing any of the listed items, it may be time for you to make some lifestyle changes, consider a different career or consider retirement.

What are your financial needs? Can't ignore this question. First, let me emphasize that I am not a financial expert. To date, I am continually educating myself regarding finances. I attend free financial lectures. I follow an online financial expert and there is still more I need to educate myself on. What I do know and recommend is that you, as early on in your career as possible, seek out a financial consultant. They will be the ones to really guide you towards your retirement goals and dreams. It's never too late, my friend.

What about your family's needs? What are your personal needs? If you have a family, it's hard to ignore how your retirement could impact them. I just caution you to remember your own needs too. Do you have family members that need more of your time and support? What are your aging parent's needs, your grandchildren? Maybe there are no outside family needs that would factor into your retirement decision but you have personal needs and concerns. If there are, write them down. Break things apart. Maybe you can't retire just yet, but you can reduce your hours. Maybe it will be obvious that others in your family need you more than your healthcare patients. Just break it down, my friend. For me, the answers usually appear when I logically collate things rather than let them play pinball in my head.

This section wouldn't be complete without sharing my thoughts on how to care and serve patients during this time of transition. This just cannot be ignored. I think we would all agree that to truly care about the welfare of our patients, we must attempt to make a smooth and gentle passage for them. If you determine retirement or a career change is in your near future, please communicate your intentions to your office manager, employer or HR department. Get everyone fully on board to help create the best transitions for everyone involved. If you don't have someone identified to take over for you, begin having different substitutes work for the day. Get your patient's feedback about that experience for them. Have your co-workers pay attention to other details that would affect their working relationship. Ultimately you may not have anything to do with the choices made to replace you, but you may have more influence than you realize. Be honest and speak up about your thoughts. And when a person is chosen, set them up for success. Remind them to be their awesome self and that you believe in them. Remind them of the routine your patients have been used to. And make sure they know you did your best serving them. It may not have been perfect, but it was your best.

So, what do you think? Are you at a place of transition or have you already arrived at your destination? Personally, I'm a little bit of both. I feel like I've only been able to share a splatter of all that I've encountered these past 40 years. A wise person once shared with me that retiring to something is much healthier than retiring from something. So, on that sweet note of advice, when my time comes, I will retire towards an active volunteer life serving others in my family and community. I hope, along the way, the love and kindness I have shared with every patient and coworker will spill out in the world. It has been pure joy. Thank you for sharing the journey with me. I will leave you with a favorite parable that I believe best describes my beautiful but cracked life.

A water bearer in India had two large pots, one hung on each end of a pole, which she carried across her neck.

One of the pots had a crack in it. While the other pot was perfect, and always delivered a full portion of water at the end of the long walk from the stream to the mistress's house, the cracked pot arrived only half full.

For a full two years, this went on daily, with the bearer delivering only one and a half pots full of water to her mistress's house.

The perfect pot was proud of its accomplishments, perfect to the end for which it was made. But the poor cracked pot was ashamed of its own imperfection and miserable that it was able to accomplish only half of what it had been made to do.

"Why?" asked the bearer. "What are you ashamed of?"

After two years of what it perceived to be a bitter failure, it spoke to the water bearer one day by the stream: "I am ashamed of myself, and I want to apologize to you."

"I have been able, for these past two years, to deliver only half my load because this crack in my side causes water to leak out all the way back to your mistress's house. Because of my flaws, you have to do all of this work, and you don't get full value from your efforts," the pot said.

The water bearer felt sorry for the old cracked pot, and in her compassion, she said, "As we return to the mistress's house, I want you to notice the beautiful flowers along the path."

Indeed, as they went up the hill, the old cracked pot took notice of the sun warming the beautiful wildflowers on the side of the path, and this cheered it some.

But at the end of the trail, it still felt bad because it had leaked out half its load, and so again it apologized to the bearer for its failure.

The bearer said to the pot, "Did you notice that there were flowers only on your side of the path, but not on the other pot's side?

"That's because I have always known about your flaw, and I took advantage of it. I planted flower seeds on your side of the path, and every day while we walk back from the stream, you've watered them.

"For two years I have been able to pick these beautiful flowers to decorate my mistress's table. Without you being just the way you are, she would not have this beauty to grace her house."

> Moral: Each of us has our own unique flaws. We're all cracked pots. But it's the cracks and flaws we each have that make our lives together so very interesting and rewarding. We've just got to take each person for what they are and look for the good in them.[22]

So, whether you identify as the water bearer, the perfect pot or the cracked pot, just remember they all played a part in the beautiful flowers growing along the path of life. You, my friend, matter and will always be enough. Thanks for sharing this part of my life's journey. My prayer is that we, together, can continue sowing seeds of compassion in this garden of life. All my best to you, always.

22 https://amazingwomenrock.com/the-cracked-pot-a-story-for-anyone-who-s-not-quite-perfect

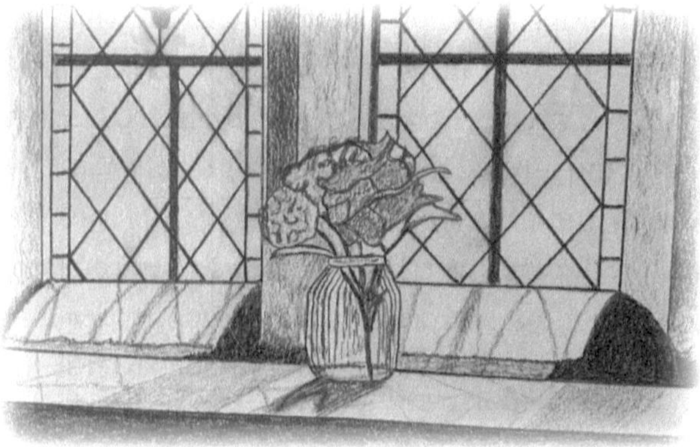

ACKNOWLEDGMENTS

With gratitude...

In my life, I've always been drawn to inspirational quotes and writings. Words that have brought me comfort, challenges, inspiration, and in some cases, a bit of wisdom. Despite all the magic a beautiful phrase has brought to me, what has most touched my soul are the relationships I've been blessed with.

Matt, Abby, Anna, Ashley, Alizabeth, Ryan and Elaine Belle. You have each been sewn into my heart. I pray you've tucked me into yours too. Thank you for the unwavering encouragement and love you have all shown me as I have moved through life. For helping me shine whatever light was inside me, out into the world. It has been through all of you, that I have most witnessed beauty, courage, devotion and the unwavering evidence of love.

Mom and Dad, your incredible examples of commitment, loyalty and love helped nourish my soul from the beginning of my life. To my mother and father-in-law, to my siblings and their families. I am so grateful for your love as well.

My dear friends who have also blessed me. To Debbie, Rachel, Judy, Terry, Deb, Jeanne and anyone else whose names have escaped my heart at this moment. You have each taught me life lessons that I will always treasure. You've all helped me grow when I didn't know how to. Thank you for your gift of friendship.

To the most incredible editor a human could be connected to, thank you, Susan. Your unending patience, encouragement and wonderful advice helped bring to print what was in my heart. A genuine thanks to John David Stein for his wonderful work and vision creating the window illustration. And, thank you Amit Dey for your patience and expertise in the typesetting process.

To every co-worker and dental patient I have been blessed to serve, a million thank yous for all the career and life lessons you taught me. Your lives have truly enriched mine. I pray I planted some seeds of love into yours as well.

To God, for his countless blessings that He has showered over me. I am so humbly grateful.

About the Author

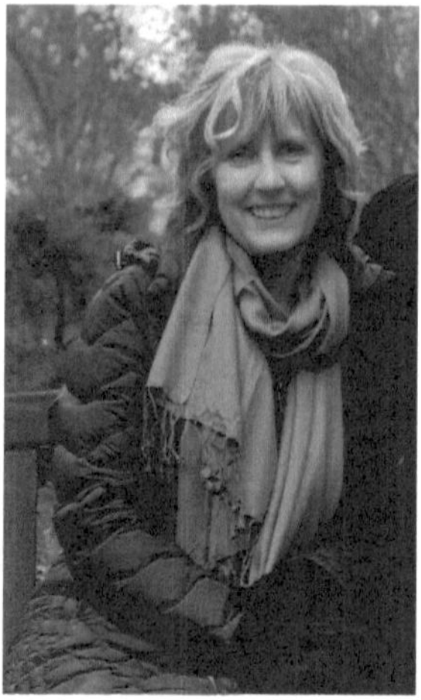

What a view it has been! Having spent over 40 years in the healthcare profession as a Registered Dental Hygienist, Judy Stein remains humble and grateful for the many blessings she has experienced. Her professional career has included invaluable opportunities in private dental practices, wonderful learning connections as a Dental Hygiene Clinical Instructor, a dream come true as a feature writer for the *RDH* magazine, co-presenter for the What Brand Are You workshop and countless hours attending continuing education classes. Whatever view Judy is looking from she does so with humbleness, a teachable heart and encouraging spirit.

She and her husband have been blessed to have helped guide four amazing daughters into this world. They reside in the gorgeous state of Michigan while also enjoying the simple joys of traveling. Judy remains active in many faith-based, community and volunteer roles. She is committed to living each day with a grateful heart, letting others know they are never alone and are always worth it!

Made in United States
Troutdale, OR
11/03/2026

56852698R10135